Soft Bipolar

Soft Bipolar

✦

Vivid Thoughts, Mood Shifts and Swings, Depression, and Anxiety of the Mild Mood Disorders Affecting Millions of Americans

Information and Help is Finally Emerging on These Misdiagnosed and Ignored Disorders

Charles K. Bunch, Ph.D.
Director of Boise Bipolar Center

iUniverse, Inc.
New York Lincoln Shanghai

Soft Bipolar
Vivid Thoughts, Mood Shifts and Swings, Depression, and Anxiety of the Mild Mood Disorders Affecting Millions of Americans

iUniverse books may be ordered through booksellers or by contacting:

iUniverse
2021 Pine Lake Road, Suite 100
Lincoln, NE 68512
www.iuniverse.com
1-800-Authors (1-800-288-4677)

ISBN-13: 978-0-595-34824-4 (pbk)
ISBN-13: 978-0-595-79555-0 (ebk)
ISBN-10: 0-595-34824-6 (pbk)
ISBN-10: 0-595-79555-2 (ebk)

Printed in the United States of America

Contents

They didn't believe you!

You felt something was not right in your head and now you will find out what the mild mood disorders (soft bipolar) are and what to do about them.

It has been confusing. Maybe there have been panic, obsessions, fear, and job problems. Things just have not turned out the way they should have. Now, there is hope, and you can rebuild and fully restart your life out from under the control of mild mood problems.

In this book, you will also find out:

- why your family physician may not be screening for the mood disorders and may be prescribing the wrong medication, which could have harmful long-term effects;

- why your psychiatrist may have ignored a diagnosis of mood disorder, and is only treating the symptoms present, delaying your recovery;

- why your therapist, although well meaning, may not be leading you to improvement;

- why incorrect or multiple mental diagnoses are harming your life.

But there is new and easy-to-understand information about the mild mood disorders. There are things you can do about this and know how to find qualified treatment in your community. And there is a place where you can help yourself to mountains of information and resources—the Internet—where up-to-date help and research on the mood disorders is a click away.

Did you know?

You could be more prone to mood disorder illnesses like those described in this book if any of these characteristics exist in your family:

alcoholism

anxiety or panic attacks

arthritic-like symptoms (fibromyalgia, chronic fatigue syndrome)

behavioral addictions or compulsions

child abuse or spousal abuse

chronic aches and pains

chronic digestive problems

chronic headaches or migraines

compulsive gambling

compulsive shopping

criminal activity and/or incarceration

depression not related to life events

drug abuse or drug addiction

eating disorders (bulimia, bingeing, or anorexia)

eccentric behavior

explosive anger/prolonged anger

hyperactivity

hypersensitivity to light, noises, touch, crowds, etc.

kleptomania

mood swings

past history of psychiatric treatment ✓

pedophilia

reactiveness/destructiveness

religious addiction or religious compulsions

seasonal depressions

self-mutilation (i.e. cutting, headbanging, and scratching)

sleep disorders

suicide or suicide threats ✓

talking continually, talking fast

tourettes disorder

unusual reactions to prescription medications

withdrawal or agoraphobia behaviors

(Adapted from "Family History Pointers to Mental Illness (Bipolar Disorder)" in http://groups.msn.com/ABipolarCommunity/familyhistory.msnw)

Do you have varying periods of:

- sharpened and creative thinking alternating with periods of mental confusion and apathy *yes*

- good mood versus times of low or irritable mood *yes*

- loss of interest or pleasure versus elevated and expansive mood *yes*

- decreased need for sleep versus too much need for sleep *yes*

- shaky self esteem and lack of self confidence versus naïve grandiose overconfidence *yes*

- unusual work hours with much done versus periods of down time and recuperation *yes*

- more uninhibited people seeking or social good times versus introverted self-absorption or withdrawal from others *no*

- involvement in pleasurable activities versus restricted involvement in pleasurable actives and feelings of guilt over past activities *no*

- optimism or exaggeration of past achievement versus pessimistic attitude toward the future or brooding about past events *yes*

- more talkative than usual with laughing, joking, and punning versus less talkative with tearfulness or crying *no*

- financial extravagance versus periods of guilt and self punishment *yes*

- more sexual or impulsive versus over-constraint or held-back *no*

- shopping, spending, and doing versus low activity *no*

- feeling in slow motion versus feeling in fast motion. *yes*

- feeling serious or morbid versus happy *yes*

- feeling like your body is heavy or you feel old versus feeling light or energetic *yes*

- feeling aware of the outer world versus feeling introspective and that others are looking at you *no*

- feeling resourceful and having ideas versus feeling stuck and limited *yes*

- having strong or increased body senses and sensations versus feeling everything is dull, tasteless, and boring   *no*

- feeling free to live in the world and society versus feeling you live in your head and are stuck with painful feelings, especially guilt and self-criticism

To Professionals and those that are Internet research savvy: why does this book take a broader view of the mood disorders than the standard diagnostic methods of the US Diagnostic Statistical Manual IV?

If you are reading this to try to assess the possibility that you or someone you treat or love might have a mood disorder, you may want to skip this section on why this book varies from some other books and diagnostic methods regarding mood disorders. However, I have included this section for both my many colleagues and a majority of Americans: the web savvy that will do their own research *now* to confirm or disprove ideas. Oh, Google, you have brought research to our very doorstep!

I have found it important in this book to broaden the definitions bipolar II and cyclothymia to allow individuals to assess less mood disorder variations and common symptoms that may indicate the presence of a treatable disorder. Also, the term cyclothymia is used in a broader sense representing a milder form of Bipolar II.

The standard of American mental disorder diagnosis is the Diagnostic Statistical Manual IV. It is used by 70% of American clinicians, including therapists, psychiatrists, and family physicians. There are those who would like a broader view of the mood disorders and find that the Diagnostic Manual falls short with limited types and rigid symptom criteria for the mood disorders.

The European view of the mood disorders is much broader and includes variations of the mood disorders, subtypes, and mild versions. Research supports this view (J Affect Disorder. 1997 May;43(3):169-80). For instance, the European view describes cyclothymic disorder as having a persistent instability of mood, involving numerous periods of mild depression and mild elation (the US view requiring hypomanic states). Cyclothymic disorder includes the milder mood disorders. The typical US view is that cyclothymic disorder is not necessarily mild. The European and an evolving US perspective allow many more individuals with mild or variational mood disorders the access to treatment. (http://mental-health.com/icd/p22-md03.html)

There are others on our continent seeking to have a more inclusive view of the mood disorders so that people who need treatment can get it. Dialogue and research is progressing on:

1. Sub-threshold bipolar types (J. Affect Disorder 2003 Jan:73(1-2): 133-46)

2. "Softer" or mild and subtle forms of the mood disorders (Bipolar Disord 2002;4 Suppl 1:11-4)

3. Investigating Bipolar ll as a full spectrum of disorders. In other words, there may be a number of Bipolar ll types that would represent a spectrum of different of these. (Psychiatr. Clin North Am 2002 Dec:25(4): 713-37). Perhaps this approach would say that cyclothymia disorder is a type of Bipolar 2.

4. Mild symptoms could be mood disorder manifestations, and these are normally missed in diagnosis. This includes the depressive temperament, melancholy episodes, and the hyperthymic temperament (J Affect Disord 1997 May;43(3):169-80)

5. Investigating all types of symptoms, including isolated symptoms where usually a whole cluster of symptoms was necessary for a diagnosis. One such effort is being done by researchers that are a part of the mood disorder Spectrum Project (http://www.namiscc.org/News/2004/Newsletters/Summer/McManVol6-20.htm)

By following strict and narrow diagnostic requirements, we fail in diagnosis and treatment:

"…by requiring the presence of both full-blown hypomanic and depressive episodes (for Bipolar ll), current nosology fails to include symptoms or signs which are mild and do not meet threshold criteria (J Affect Disord 1999 Aug;54(3) :319-28).

And in practice, prestigious research and treatment facilities and professionals are expanding definitions. Massachusetts General Hospital Bipolar Clinic and Research Program uses Bipolar lll, although this in not included in the American Diagnostic Manual lV.

…it is a useful concept. In our clinic, the diagnosis is used for a person who has recurrent Major Depressive Episodes, and has never had an elevated mood episode. This person does, however, have a parent, child or sibling that meets the criteria for Bipolar l Disorder, Bipolar ll Disorder, or Cyclothymia (cyclothymic disorder)." (http://www.manicdepressive.org/dsm.html)

There is a case for cyclothymia being a milder form of Bipolar ll. There are professional case studies:

"Here is an example. Ariel, a 16-year-old girl, had a history of repeated severe suicidal depressions punctuated by periods of a few hours, sometimes a day or two (definitely not four days as prescribed in the Diagnostic and Statistical Manual of Mental Disorders, Fourth Edition for hypomania), in which she felt a bit goofy as well as more social, energetic and creative. There was no family history of manic-depressive illness. She did not feel that her "up" times were a problem. Indeed, she was able to perform a high level academically and felt more connected to her friends and parents. There was no pressured speech, flight of ideas or a sense that her mind was racing. There was no distractibility, impulsivity, irresponsible spending, driving or sexual behavior, or loss of judgment. Insomnia was not present, and there was not history of a decreased need for sleep. Although there was an improvement in self-esteem, it was not inflated or grandiose. Ariel's parents and friends, as well as Ariel herself considered her good mood entirely normal and delighted in them.

Ariel did have "mood swings." She would be in a perfectly good mood and then suddenly, with relatively minor provocation, switch to sadness, irritability or an outburst of anger. This was the other major justification for placement on a "mood stabilizer." There's only one problem with this. The use of the term mood swings in bipolar disorder has usually referred not to labile (changing) affect, but to relatively long stretches of depression or mania lasting weeks or month-although occasionally days-which would then swing to the opposite." (http://psycyhiatrictimes.com/p991036.html)

There is support that cyclothymia is a milder mood disorder. Some are impaired by the disorder. But for others, "They are not impaired with the high…they're facilitated by it. If the depression is not too debilitating, they function better than average." In this same article, the author Debra Wood, RN supports a broad trigger cause of mood shift. Some professionals stand firm on their view that mood shifts are caused "spontaneously" or independent of internal or external cues (such as stress). The author points out that stress and life events are causes of mood shifting. (http://healthinfo.healthgate.com, The Ups and Downs of Cyclothymia)

Unipolar Depression (depression with no up mood state) is thought to be a form of the mood disorders and not just depression. It is a distinguishable form of depression and is not validated in the DSM-IV:

"Eight years is an eternity when it comes to getting the correct diagnosis, much less the appropriate treatment. Fortunately, reading between the lines of the DSM-VI(nci) Code can speed up the process. One means is to closely prove individual depression for "unipolar" or 'bipolar" characteristics. In a study of separate unipolar and bipolar populations comprising 493 patients, Dr. Akiskal and Nantouche teased out a number of distinguishing features, namely:

Those with bipolar II depression experienced greater suicidal thinking, guilt, depersonalization, and derealization. Despite hypersomnia and weight gain, they experience more psychomotor activation, suggesting a missed depressive state.

Patients with unipolar depression, on the other hand, had a more psychic anxiety and insomnia, and rated high on slow thinking, lack of energy, feeling worst, avoiding risks, life dull, and dreary.

Needless to say, the above distinctions may entirely elude many clinicians. Accordingly, in another article, Dr. Akiskal proposes the following behavioral characteristics, based on his own clinical experience:

Proficiency in three or more languages (which is rare amongst people in the US but may not apply in Europe), working in fields that require personal charm and eloquence such as diplomacy, journalism, and entertainment; creativity (especially those who excel in three or more domains); instability in life (such as going to three universities without getting a degree or changing professions from one to another to yet another); activity junkies (such as individuals who travel long distances more than three times a month); substance use (especially three or more drugs); co-occurring illnesses (such as those with at least three anxiety disorders); multiple outrageous behaviors (including borderline personality, compulsive gambling, sexual addition, and taking extreme risks); sexual excesses; flamboyance (such as pink socks in a male patient).

...Dr. Akiskal does not suggest slapping a bipolar label on every engaging and creative individual who just happens to look stunning in Versace, but he does urge that clinicians be mindful of the warning signs and carefully screen these patients for bipolar (http://www.namiscc.org/News/2005/Newsletters/WinterMcManVol7-5.htm)

It is not only important to look at soft bipolar types, but to also look at bipolar symptoms or mild types as precursors of more severe types. (same reference as above). Obviously, early treatment of a mild cyclothymic disorder makes sense especially if it prevents Bipolar l or ll from opening up.

Other types of soft bipolars are considered that do not fit the usual categories:

1. There are those with depressed mixed states where mixed state has often been thought of related to an up state (mixed mania) or just a transition from one mood to another (Am J Psychiatry 162:193-194, January 2005).

2. There are very angry mixed-states documented (http://angelfire3.com/home/bphoenix1/mixed.html)

3. There are particularly irritable depresseds that are ignored by DSM-lV for a mood disorder diagnosis (http://www.mcmanweb.com/mood_spectrum.htm)

So why is all this so important? By not having a broader view of the symptoms and diagnosis of the mood disorders, including soft types, several things happen:

1. Obviously, those who need current treatment are not given access to that because they are not diagnosed as such.

2. Those who have precursor symptoms such as depression, or self-mediation with drugs or alcohol are also skipped

3. Patients are often given a mis-diagnose and resulting wrong medications and therapies

4. There is loss of quality of life for the individual who is not treated. Because of this, society and even the economy do not have the benefit of having a fully functional individual.

5. Time and patient money is lost

    "The clinical stakes, however, are such that a narrow concept of bipolar disorder would deprive many patients with a lifelong temperamental dysregulation and depressive episodes the benefits of mood-regulating agents." (J. Clin. Pharmacol 1996 Apr;16(2Suppl_1):45-145)

6. To not have good information on this promotes public ignorance. In one case I noticed, a patient with pain and rapid mood shifts stated his case in an internet support group posting. Although at least one person suggested an accurate diagnosis of cyclothymic disorder based on the symptoms, many postings suggest he had other disorders, including poisoning from mercury dental fillings. In this case the patient could not only evade appropriate treatment but also go down some costly erroneous other path. He stated that he made a commitment to see an expensive specialist to have his fillings all replaced to alleviate his "mercury poisoning".

So, you can see that others are seeking to broaden the definitions of the mood disorders to include the soft types. Patients and our communities at large are benefited from this. In my clinical practice, I have noticed that these ideas put into practice result in positive outcomes: people are diagnosed, treated, and have tremendously improved lives. That's what counts most.

Please note: in this book, Bipolar l, ll, lll, and so on were designated as 1, 2, 3, and so on. My patients suggested this to make the terms understandable for the general population for whom this book is intended for.

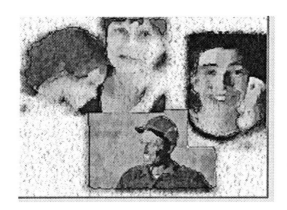

References: This is a book for the average person on the street, someone who wants information for personal help. So, in this technological age, the Internet is now our library. For that reason, I am providing more "reader friendly" references that include the web site address for the reference. I hope that this manner of reference encourages your own referral to that particular site.

While bipolar mood disorder is often listed into different types with Roman Numerals (Bipolar l, ll, and lll, etc.), we are using regular numbers (Bipolar 1, 2, and 3).

Acknowledgments

I would like to thank these folks for all their personal support: my dad Bert, a fount of wisdom and information, Martina Saffron, Shannon and Neil Fausey (who kindly developed my website www.MoodDisorder.net), Roberto and Beth Leoni and Lucas Resende of Brazil.

To, Bethe Hagens, Ph.D., I always find some small piece of inspiration around my house that was a result of your help in my doctoral studies at the Union Institute and University.

There are many new physicians, therapists, and trainers out there that are creating a new world for mood disorder sufferers. My hat goes off to them. Scott Hoopes, M.D., thanks for information and encouragement. I have also found a vital side to the pharmaceutical companies: treating bipolar disorder well is their passion, and their many representatives have made important resources available to me. I especially thank Kris Samer of Abbott Laboratories (makers of Depakote).

Thanks Leah Hopkins, managing editor of the *Messenger Index* newspaper, for technical editing at inconvenient times. Jon, Curtis, and Greg, your comments were critical for this book.

Lastly, I have learned much from my patients themselves. They have allowed me to share a bit of their journey and struggle with the mood disorders. These persons do not just have a brain disorder, but great depth of soul and breadth of knowledge that makes the world richer.

1

A personal introduction: Why I do this

Originally, materials were needed urgently for my own patients, to validate the pain of misdiagnosis and their problems. There just seemed to be no reliable materials that provided up-to-date clinical information that was readily understandable. My patients were just sitting ducks when they went into a doctor's office to discuss their mood problem.

These people needed more than my opinion; they needed terms, charts, solid research, courage, armor, and maybe some weapons in hand. Too many were becoming victims of psychiatric and psychological mistakes and were paying the price through years of incorrect treatment and residual suffering. It had to stop and I told them so.

I am glad to say that there are many people who now call, write, and drop by to thank me for helping get them on the right track—a different track:

- a track of more self-sufficiency and knowledge

- a track of more collaborative direction in their treatment of a mood disorder with their treatment providers

- a track of fewer wrong medications that stem from a wrong diagnosis

- a track where there is validation for the suffering and an understanding of the life risks of the mild mood disorders

- a track where there are things each person can do, in addition to taking correct mood stabilizer medication, that can greatly reduce mood shifting

- a track where you can finally put vivid thoughts and feelings, mood swings, and depression in perspective so that this soft bipolar mood problem is manageable

I love working in the field of mood disorder treatment

I'm the greatest mood disorder magnet in the world. I can pick them out in any crowd. All my best friends have some sort of mood disorder and many take some form of medication for it. I really like these folks as they're not known as the "salt of the earth" types; they are the "spice of life" types. They bring seasoning to the world.

Most all of us have painful moods and anxiety and most humans suffer at some point in their lives. It is just that we grab for the wrong treatments for them: booze, carbohydrates, escapism, anger, or any other outlet.

Personally, I was fortunate, starting as a mental health counselor 20 years ago, to be influenced by a person who loved to treat his mood disorder patients. This psychiatrist felt that mild depression and many anxiety disorders were probably hidden mood disorders (then called manic-depressive illness). To his credit, he had many successes.

Then, I began many years of structured outpatient treatment with many challenging clients who had complex problems with panic attacks, social phobias, obsessive-compulsive disorder, and mild depression. These complex disorders caused personal, work, and marriage problems.

Usually, these individuals have seen many therapists and many psychiatrists over the years without making any headway. Eventually, observable patterns emerged. There were:

- family patterns of undiagnosed mild mood disorders that were often missed by common diagnostic methods or by their mental health professionals

- patterns of switching into mild mania when starting or taking antidepressants

- bubbly and overly active moods seen as a good sign rather than a part of mood cycles

- patients who could not get validation or supportive materials because some had mild mood disorders that were either only borderline noticeable or covered up with other symptoms, other medical problems, or personal problem

- treatment influenced by medications that were highly marketed (there was the Prozac era, the Zoloft era, etc.)

- therapy with not enough information to patients, and physicians not knowing that therapy assisted the medications in working on the brain disorder, called bipolar mood disorder

Over the years, I have spent countless hours studying bipolar treatment and always enjoyed it. I have become a bipolar observer. The more I learn about this, the more I pick up bipolar symptom clues from others in their normal walks of life: a depressed person in the corner of a coffeehouse, a bubbly person being the life of the party, or some talking a million miles an hour about some new project they've started or dreamed of.

To Describe

To be able to describe something gives us a sense of understanding and greater control in seemingly uncontrollable situations. We have struggles with what to call the milder mood disorders that are not bipolar 1.

Are they part of a spectrum of mood disorders?

Are they soft bipolar because they're mild versions of bipolar l?

Maybe they are just variations of bipolar l.

Should there be a bipolar 2, 3, 4, etc. to describe many types?

I like the term soft bipolar, which includes the milder mood disorders that will be described later: bipolar 2 and bipolar 3 cyclothymic disorder. It is not fully settled what these will be called. But by describing them, we will certainly come up with agreed upon names and classifications of the mild moods.

Do you have any ideas, comments, or suggestions on the soft bipolar? Please forward your comments or questions to me at cbunchphd@MoodDisorder.net, and we will all learn more together.

While several authors state that six to nine percent of the population suffers from mood disorders, I will keep it very conservative here. Still, if we say that three percent of the American population suffers, that is nine-million individuals. You are in good company.

More about the Author

Dr. Bunch completed his Master's Degree in mental health counseling at Idaho State University, and his attained his doctorate in Counseling from the Union Institute and University in Cincinnati, Ohio. He is a Licensed Clinical Counselor and National Certified Counselor in clinical practice in Boise Idaho.

Dr. Bunch has spoken in the US and overseas on topics of depression, panic, phobias, mood disorders, communication, sex and sexuality, and many other topics. He has run structured treatment programs for the treatment of agoraphobia, obsessive-compulsive disorder, and substance abuse. As a Jungian therapist, Dr. Bunch has completed e-books on metaphor therapy, cinematherapy, and working with metaphoric mind monsters.

He has also completed extensive studies on world culture, myth, and the place of spirituality and faith in each person's health process. Here are two favorite quotations of Dr. Bunch:

> *Our deepest fear is not that we are inadequate. Our deepest fear is that we are powerful beyond measure.*
>
> —Marianne Williamson

This quote is originally from Marianne Williamson and later quoted by Nelson Mandela at his inauguration.

> *Keep knocking, and the joy inside will eventually open a window and look outside to see who's there.*
>
> —Rumi (a 13th century Sufi poet)

2

More than just friendly, more than just bubbly

Did you see the movie or TV shows Dragnet? The prologue always said that "what you are about to see is a true story, but the details have been changed to protect the innocent." So, too, the basics of the stories in this book are all true. But, any details that would link them to a real person have been changed to protect privacy.

With that in mind:

Jane was a neighbor I lived next door to for 10 years. I got to know her pretty well over that time as we lived on the same cul-de-sac. Most times, she was bubbly, showing up with a friend in her car, stuffing me in at the last minute to go to a restaurant. She was the life of the party. You could see heads turn as her smile drew attention from all around.

But I did know the other side of that bubbly person. She would come over and walk in without knocking and "helpfully" push her way around the kitchen. It was all well intentioned. Even if you'd planned a quiet evening, she'd have you making homemade pasta and bread in no time.

Life was a party, and you were mostly better for it, she thought. I learned early on not to criticize this, as she would become instantly offended. A big outburst of tears would follow. Happy would turn to sobbing. With the fun was a lot of other emotionality.

But there was an even darker side of Jane. Throughout the year, she had "spells," during which she said she just could not move. She said she was just worn out, exhausted. Eventually, I recognized this as the down side of her "up." She would lounge around in her pajamas. She felt her arms and legs were heavy.

I noticed cleaning in the house would go undone for days with smelly dishes piling up. She complained that the mail was a project that "burdened" her, an awful, heavy project she just could not get to.

Suddenly, the happy-go-lucky-person had switched. It wasn't really awful because, over time, she would move out of this. The problem, though, was that her ob-gyn started to note these down spells in regular check-ups and assumed that this was simple depression. And, even worse, a trial of Paxil perked up Jane in two days and the doctor felt overly pleased with of that.

Jane started on what she started to call the Paxil Roller Coaster. She was up for a couple of weeks when she started the medication, but eventually this led to depression and stopping Paxil. Soon, there would be another shot at the medication, as Jane got accustomed to the restart period. Again, for a while, she could be bubbly and overly productive. A dirty house soon smelled of Lysol cleaner.

Jane was starting into more severe mood cycles. She was not just the bubbly person. There was more:

- aggression: she was always intrusive, but now there was a bit meanness to it

- uninhibited times where she would blurt things out without reservation

- times where she was just "off the wall" in some odd flighty mode

- scatteredness

- less fun

- rapidly changing moods

- anxiety and fear

Jane went through several of these cycles of Paxil. Finally, her own intuition kicked in, and she decided to go off the antidepressant "cold turkey." However, she eventually moved into a long-term depression that had more severe problems: problems thinking and with thoughts, lower mood, and guilt. Not just her personal life but also her work life was now impacted.

Jane had gone from simple mood swings to severe anxiety and depression. She was a "mixed bag" of symptoms now.

She moved away for a new job, feeling that escape from the current geographic setting might help. But the basis for change should have been starting appropriate mood stabilizers.

This is a typical scenario for mild mood disorder.

> We are using the terms soft bipolar and mild mood disorder somewhat interchangeably in this book. By mild, we mean milder than the most noted mood disorder, bipolar 1, described briefly below. While I sometimes use the term mild moods or mild mood disorders, my patients have preferred the idea of "soft bipolar." Most have told me that while this is not bipolar 1, there is nothing really mild about it. In fact, it can be pretty torturous.

Soft bipolar sufferers are very likely to be misdiagnosed. The consequences can be severe, ranging from lost quality of life to suicidal thoughts.

What the public thinks of as "classic bipolar disorder" is bipolar 1

While this book does not focus on the most commonly known form of bipolar disorder—manic depression (or bipolar 1),—we do need to mention it. It is the big, beefy, and most commonly recognized, brother of the mild mood disorder. Some treatment specialists feel that, if untreated, or treated incorrectly, mild mood disorders can progress to this more severe form. Certainly, soft bipolar persons who have done or do illicit drugs can be diagnosed as bipolar 1.

Since we know so much about bipolar 1, we can benefit from the wealth of knowledge available. Even though all medications used to treat bipolar 1 are also effective in treating mild mood disorders, I find that counseling and educational treatment for soft bipolar needs to be distinctly different.

It was once thought that all bipolar mood disorder sufferers fit into one "mold." Formerly referred to as manic-depressive disorder, this "classic form"—alternating periods of mania and severe depression—is now called bipolar 1. Individuals can have manic (up) phases of months or years and depressed (down) phases of months or years. But there are those who can "cycle" through moods every few minutes.

Manic periods can be severe: taking extreme risks, euphoria, psychosis, extreme spending, many ideas and rapid thoughts. Depressed periods can be very dark, to the point of suicide attempts.

Bipolar 1 is a very serious disorder. These sufferers often have frequent psychiatric hospital admissions and often take multiple medications. Forty percent attempt suicide and twenty percent complete suicide.

Many famous people suffered from bipolar 1 and there are movies that document their mania, including *Amadeus, Marques De Sade,* and *Total Eclipse.*
Here is a brief list:

Writers

Hans Christian Anderson

Ernest Hemingway

Hermann Hess

Samuel Clemens (Mark Twain)

Charles Dickens

Ralph Waldo Emerson

Virginia Woolf

Famous Musicians

Handel

Mahler

Tchaikovsky

Kurt Cobain

Poets

Lord Byron

T.S. Elliot

Emily Dickinson

Ezra Pound

Walt Whitman

Edgar Allen Poe

Famous Artists

Gauguin

Van Gogh

Munch

Georgia O'Keefe

And, as mentioned in her new book, Jane Pauley.

(See page after page at <u>http://www.pendulum.org/information/</u> <u>information_famous.html</u>) And, see the book, *Touched by Fire: Manic-Depressive Illness and the Artistic* by Kay Redfield Jamison)

Are there any famous soft bipolar persons? I am sure there are many, but since their stories are not so distinct and they function better in life, we won't know of many of them. I often speculate, based on vivid thoughts, whether many current authors or creative movie producers are soft bipolars. If so, they would lead lives with more consistent productivity than the listed bipolar ls.

I have read about the "ecstatic mystical poets" in the book, *The Soul In Love: Classic Poems of Ecstasy and Exaltation (of) Rumi, Hafiz, Kabir, Mirabai, and Tagor* by Deepak Chopra. I feel that these very emotional poets were likely soft bipolar. Again, they had ongoing productivity. Rumi composed tens of thousands of poems.

We have learned some interesting things abut bipolar 1:

- Half of bipolars are not treated. Many are homeless.

- Bipolar patients are often arrested due to bipolar behavior.

- Men and women are equally susceptible to the illness.

- There are regional and world differences in the illness and this is not fully understood. There are lower rates of the illness in Mexico and among Hutterites and the Amish.

- Bipolar disorder has direct patient and indirect social costs to American society of $45 billion per year. (<u>http://silk.nih.gov/silk/NB/papers/costmd05.html</u>).

- Bipolar disorder was less common in the nineteenth century and is becoming more prevalent now. One percent experiences bipolar l and about three to six percent experience other forms of bipolar disorder (bipolar 2 and 3).

- Bipolar disorder is a chronic brain disorder. At least five chemical components have been discovered that are related to the disorder and scientist estimate there may be as many as 20 chemical components to this.

- Bipolar is more prevalent in winter-born children.

- One-fourth of depressed patients are actually unipolar-bipolar, and have not been appropriately diagnosed as bipolar disorder. (unipolar, meaning is has one up or down pole, such as just depressed but never manic)

- One-fifth of post-partum depression and post-partum psychosis is actually bipolar disorder.

- It is generally accepted that bipolar disorder is hereditary. It is generally accepted that bipolar disorder is associated with family patterns of alcoholism and other addictions.

- Not screening depressed patients for bipolar disorder and prescribing "SSRI" antidepressants can lead to mania and long-term brain tissue damage. The SSRI medications include Prozac, Paxil, Luvox, Zoloft, and more.

- Bipolar disorder may show up in children in different forms, especially as hyperactivity. It is often misdiagnosed as attention deficit hyperactive disorder (ADHD), or more commonly as childhood depression. In fact, childhood depression may be the first indicator of a bipolar condition that may not be recognized until the person is well into their twenties or thirties. bipolar disorder in children is called COPD or child onset bipolar disorder. Specialists are able to differentiate these disorders today.

- Mood disorders can lie dormant and be "cracked" open by life events, the use of drugs, a pregnancy, etc. These are called "activating events."

While there are many books and web sites suggesting you can control mood disorders through self-help or with holistic medications, only the mood stabilizers, alone or with therapy, are proven to help control the disorders.

Sixty percent of bipolar sufferers will have a substance abuse problem at some time in their life. Substance abuse is the number-one factor contributing to medications not working well in bipolar patients.

While there are new advances and very technical medications that stabilize moods for bipolar patients, there are also low-cost, generic medications with minimal side effects.

As medications advance, there is less patient resistance to taking medications due to decreased side effects.

My perspective and that of this book, are certainly from the bipolar therapist's chair. I provide supportive and educational therapy for patients seeing a psychiatrist and taking mood-stabilizing medications. You can find ways to "get along" with soft bipolar.

While I have included some links to information on medication, we can look forward to many new, helpful books from the perspective of the mood disorder psychiatrist or pharmacologist—those working specifically with the mood stabilizing medications.

3

Diagnosis problems

Soft bipolar is not difficult to diagnose, but you have to know disorder and human issues to find it.

John's story

John came in to ask me if he could join my panic management class. He was already seeing a psychiatrist and therapist and had seen dozens of others. He had a list of diagnoses that brought a sense of despair to his face as he recounted them with shame. He was taking Paxil, Anafranil, and Zanax, which he stated was for multiple diagnoses of panic, depression and obsessive-compulsiveness disorder. John felt that over time he was becoming more of a "mental patient" and said he was even feeling worse in his head and body on this medication.

I assessed John using my Mood Disorder Screening Tool (at the end of this book) and told him I did not think I could let him into the group because he wasn't yet appropriate for the group and that his medication might be a part of the problem. I thought he might be upset with this. But he said he knew, despite what others told him that he had not yet been properly diagnosed.

John then began to accept a new diagnosis: a mild mood disorder. He then accepted a referral to a mood disorder psychiatrist who corroborated the diagnosis and prescribed medication. In time, with adjunctive outpatient therapy, he saw improvement, although some symptoms remained. But he also attained levels of independence from the mental health system that he never thought would be attainable. I, too, was pleased.

You would think it would be an easy matter to screen and treat individuals for mood disorders and even the Mild Moods, but it is not. Not only has it taken us until today to begin to label them, there are many factors that impede diagnosis and treatment.

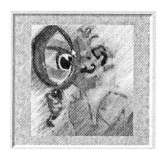

Pieces of the Puzzle

The brain is not easy to diagnose: it presents to us mental symptoms, instead of some visible wound we have to rely on while evaluating our thoughts and feelings. Soon, however, it will be more common to examine the brain via chemical scanning methods to detect anomalies caused by psychiatric disorders (which are now called brain disorders).

We will discuss some of the many problems of diagnosis in this chapter. Besides the brain being difficult to diagnose, treatment specialists (primary care physicians, psychiatrists, and therapists) may have preconceived notions. They may actually have some "preferred" disorder, or a bias to diagnose in a particular way. It is common that there is a lack of knowledge about how to screen for or properly recognize a mood disorder.

Then, there are many patient problems. Dealing with thoughts and feelings can be confusing. We may lack awareness of the problem and not be able to communicate about an odd group of symptoms.

Add to this further problems sufferers face: it often just feels normal. And, not all symptoms are seen as bad: to be buzzing around doing several projects and extremely social is seen as ok. Who really would want to stop euphoric feelings?

In addition to all this, there are actual diagnostic difficulties that have not been standardized in the treatment community in diagnosing mood disorders and in differentiating them from other psychiatric disorders.

Is bipolar diagnosis now overdone?

Some say that there is a current trend to over-diagnose mood disorders because it is just "popular." However, research is shows this to be untrue. Mood disorders are continually under-diagnosed. People suffer. And we all pay.

Early screening, diagnosis, and treatment are essential for mood disorders. We should aggressively seek to uncover the mood disorders and aggressively treat them. Otherwise, there are great risks of loss of jobs, relationships, and lives. (Please see the important article on this, Is Bipolar Disorder Misdiagnosed? by S. Nassir Ghaemi, MD at www.mhsource.com).

Most often, like John, above, patients get "backed into a diagnosis." This refers to going through years of trial and error diagnosis and treatment. Finally, at the end, a correct diagnosis might be reached. Through lots of bumps, bruises, and wrong diagnoses, they hopefully get to the correct diagnosis of a mood disorder.

But what if it took you two years or even ten years to get the correct treatment started? You could go through hell, get deeply entrenched in the mental health system, and simply lose that period of time in your life. That's bad. Not only this, the disorder-driven choices made during this period can have consequences extending years or decades beyond successful treatment (such as bankruptcy, divorce, sexually transmitted diseases, further brain damage (the "kindling effect) drug and alcohol addictions, and so on). We've got to do better and the system of "backing into a diagnosis" has got to go!

Human problems with diagnosis: What, me have a problem?

If professionals can't assess a set of symptoms, we should not expect any patient chime up and say out of the blue, "Maybe I have soft bipolar, a mild mood disorder, Cyclothymia, or *something*." There just isn't enough good information out there and it just isn't something you see on TV or in the movies

So, patients will go into the doctor's or therapist's office with a set of complaints, but they could be very, very, very skewed:

They could complain of symptoms that could be direct clues of the mood disorders: mania, behavioral problems, depression, feeling sad, lethargic, or hopeless.

Usually, though, they bring in a set of common symptoms that could also be seen as one of many psychiatric disorders: depression, panic, obsessive-compulsiveness, general anxiety, sleep problems, workaholism, alcoholism, etc.

But they might have other odd symptoms that are confusing, such as nightmares, extreme fears, day visions, fogginess, social phobias, memory problems, hyperactivity, concentration problems, oversensitivity to sound, racing thoughts, feelings of deep guilt for no apparent reason, tumultuous personal relationships, serial divorces, forgetting to eat or sleep, or agoraphobia (fear of being away from a safe place or person). Or they may be only aware of another level of problems: work, relationship, communication, or family problems.

Certainly, we tend to not to complain of feeling good or bubbly. This too can be a sign of the mood disorders. You are going to have to put on your Sherlock Holmes hat and pull out your calabash pipe for some of the mild mood disorders:

Joan had a series of mild depression problems in adulthood, but she seemed calm, normal, and reasonably pleasant. She did have a period of post-partum psychosis after the birth of her first daughter. And she reported having horrible nightmares and sometimes, vivid daytime "nightmares" that caused panic attacks. She does get overstimulated by noise and sometimes needs to withdraw. Other than this, Joan seems like about the most normal patient you ever could have met. However, in Joan's family are two bipolar brothers who have had various hospitalizations. Based on this, Joan's family physician was willing to try a mild dose of a mood stabilizer, the type her brothers take. It has worked wonders, lessening both the overall symptoms and the need for extensive counseling sessions.

Awareness and motivation

It is estimated that among all bipolar patients, 40 percent do not have insight into their problem. It is not a bad thing, or their choice to not recognize this. The brain does not deliver the message that there is a problem here. It is like putting a frog in a pan of water and slowly, slowly turning on the heat. The frog is oblivious to the increasing problem and will stay in the hot water until death.

The soft bipolars, the mild moods, will continue in the mood states, not knowing that it may be dysfunctional. Lack of awareness can be a problem, but if you are aware, lack of motivation can also be a problem. After you have had a Mild Mood for many years, you can become attached to it. Take a look at these examples:

Depressed Mom, sad, withdrawn, has learned to safely watch TV for many years, and to change this would be too threatening.

Mildly manic Mary gets lots of attention for her smile. What would she do if she were not such a socialite?

Anxious Juan has run his life on dealing with various depressive and anxious states. He attends several support groups. He might feel lost without having support groups to meet people and use personal time.

Workaholic businessman Joe wouldn't be able to function at his accustomed high level if he were to treat the hypomania.

When we become hooked on some dysfunctional routine in our life that is not too awful, but not the best we could do, we call this an "ego attachment."

Through medication and treatment, mood disorder sufferers often find they can rebuild a second life after recovery. A great book to help with this is *A Setback is a Setup for a Comeback* by Willie Jolley, a book full of affirmations on rebuilding one's life.

Mild moods don't always look like a disorder

It's easy to tell many Bipolar 1s on first glance if they are not medicated. They might be talking rapidly and will not allow interruption, or if they are a psychotic type, even talking to someone or something else.

But this is not the case with soft bipolar. If you saw them at the state fair, they might not stand out more than any other person. If you got to know them better, you would find them (according to their sub-type) to have some ongoing or consistent characteristics that may or may not be associated with mood swinging. Maybe you've met someone like this:

- A person you take to movies who often makes a scene over emotional parts of a movie. For instance, there might be notable episodes of strong weeping, crying, or sobbing and you are embarrassed to be with that person.

- The aunt who gets too involved in telling old stories. Some mild moods just have too much sentimentality or emotionality.

- The friend who can always make it to work but seems mildly depressed. Perhaps this person is overly is quiet or withdrawn. They could talk in whispers. Possibly that have little social life outside of work.

- The secret or subtle mood shifter. Periods of mental collapse or heaviness following activity no one knows about; may even disappear for a few days.

- The adult child of a bipolar 1. This is the pushy and aggressive person who has few other symptoms. Hmmm, is he or she is working on the sixth rocky marriage?

- The crude dad who will eventually put all his kids in "therapy". Dad can be pretty friendly at work, but his kids know the dark side of dad—volatile, moody, snappy, and never has a nice thing to say at home.

- The fearful. This person keeps her family busy with her fears, has periods of panic, fear, social phobia, and almost paranoia.

- The person who always "up" or grandiose about life.

- Those without social boundaries. There are those who are just too helpful.

- The overly emotional person who can also be destructive and abusive. One wife throws fits, throws plates and furniture. The police are called, but oddly the behavior is just "excused" as a marital problem. The woman is allowed to continue a life of extreme emotions and behavior.

- Confusing patterns tiredness, tardiness, or missing work. The exuberant person you hired, who seemed totally competent, flops a few days later.

- The neighborhood kid, with good grades at school who just seems a little "dark" in manner. Who would know that that dark troubling brilliance is part of a mood disorder?

Sometimes, a hunch or gut feeling helps

I feel much wiser now having treated many soft bipolars. For instance, I have run a Fearful Flyers' Clinic for many years, to assist those persons in overcoming the fear of getting on jets. We all like to take vacations, handle business trips, or need to go a funeral. For some, this generates severe anxiety and visions of tragedy.

But I know now how deep and visceral fears can be for mood disorder sufferers. I no longer just give fearful mood disorder sufferers the short class and then the goodbye at the plane with my parting words "you'll be fine." I now spend much more time coaching them on how to contain the very visually oriented images their creative imagination generates. These can be terrifying images that seem like complete pictures or movie. Some feel they are so real that they are premonitions of something about to occur.

Henrique was asked by his employer to participate in a "ropes course." In this ropes course, his work team would develop personal and teamwork skills while traversing a series of ropes in trees at a mountain retreat. This was like a jungle gym course of ropes strung high in pine trees. Just telling me about the planned event made Henrique turn white!

He had just been properly diagnosed and had only been on medication for a few days. I assured Henrique that all the talking in the world would not help him prepare for the event coming up in two weeks, and that emergency tranquilizers could be dangerous.

Since Henrique did not want to have his employer get a letter from his "therapist," we arranged for his physician to give him a letter stating that he could not attend the event for "some medical" reason, which more than satisfied his employer. In subsequent meetings, Henrique was able to understand and begin to work with his very visceral fears as well as communicate these symptoms to his doctor to gear his medications in this treatment route.

We are looking at symptoms that taken individually can look normal, but very illuminating when observed as a set. What is wrong with being emotional, happy, or any other characteristic of the mild moods? Nothing. There is nothing wrong with each on its own. But added up, these symptoms are they diagnostic clues for the mood disorders.

So, why are people not diagnosed correctly? Certainly, there are those treatment specialists (doctors and therapists) who do not know or are not interested in screening or diagnosing the mood disorders. But, with the mood disorders, we have to look at several factors and not just the set of symptoms presented to a doctor (simply called the presenting symptoms).

Diagnosis needs to be:

- comprehensive—covering broadly, completely, inclusively.

- longitudinal—dealing with the growth, change, and period of years of the person (i.e. it is historical).

- contextual—looking at how the person functions in the context of their life, job, relationships, etc.

Here is a chart comparing the different characteristics of the two diagnosis methods and comparisons:

Historical, Comprehensive, and Contextual Diagnosis	Symptom-Only Based Diagnosis
based on historical view and the present set of symptoms	based on a present symptom
looks at the patient's and the family's medical or psychological history—This can include prior diagnoses in relatives or looking at symptoms observed in relatives (for instance, "Dad was pretty moody, but never treated for that" "Aunt Mabel was eccentric.")	looks just at the patient in the office
Looks at historical responses and current responses to medications as further clues to diagnosis	may actually increase medication or add a similar medication if the existing medication is not working

driven to find a diagnosis for an overall disorder	seeks to remove a set of symptoms present today regardless of patterns or harm done
gathers feedback from other treatment specialists, family members, etc.	again, looks at present symptoms only; does not include the reports of others

We should look at:

Life history—A personal mood, depression, and anxiety history is reviewed.

The Longitudinal Life History is a long-term historical view of your life, to detect patterns of periods of depression, mild mania, and any other symptoms. Any personal historical and medical materials compiled on this helps, but often, a "life timeline" drawn out on a large piece of paper is most helpful. This is a long line with all your birth dates, major life events, and medical events posted on it.

You would include on this the starting and stopping of any medications. Throw in any serious life stressor such as school, work issues, death in the family, etc. If a person can, attempts at noting periods of mood states, anxiety and depression are included.

All prior diagnoses—Often, patients have been told by prior professionals that personality disorders, eating disorders, or a mood disorder "might be suspected."

Response to all prior medications—This is a list of all psychotropic medications. This class of medications includes the antidepressants, tranquilizers, stimulants, mood stabilizers, and antipsychotics.

Family history (called "pedigree")—The most helpful tool for the pedigree is the family tree. Draw out the tree of your brothers and sisters, parents, aunts, uncles, etc. Then, list all known biological disorders of each. Then, add any characteristics about each person, including anxiety, panic, attention problems, eccentric or odd behavior, drinking, drugs, behavior problems, legal problems, money problems, marital problems, anger, moody, happy, depressed, withdrawn, etc.

Current symptoms—recent, and those of the last year, including secondary disorders (such as panic attacks, attention problems, etc.).

Other medical issues—There are many other medical disorders that can mimic psychiatric disorders (anxiety, depression, the mood disorders, and so on). This includes thyroid problems, neurological problems, and drug-induced mania or depression.

Included at the end of the book is a Mood Disorder Screening Tool, which covers some of the basics of the mood disorders. Unlike others I have found, it includes symptoms for both bipolar 1 and soft bipolar.

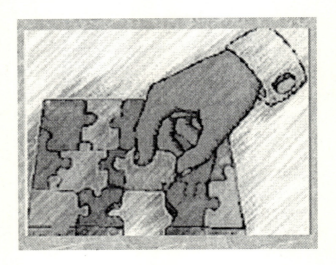

4

Core thought factors of soft bipolar

There are several psychological elements that are common to the mild moods and bipolar 1. They come from both biology and thinking. The issues listed are not exclusive to the mood disorders. However, they are more extreme if you have a mood disorder.

Vivid and Florid Thoughts

Laksmi shared concern that she kept a secret from others. When coming across different people, she would often fixate on some facial feature of a person. She then found the feature, such as a bent nose, quirky eyebrows, etc., to be disgusting. But, her mind quickly went to repulsion—to the point that she felt the person was grotesque or frightening.

Laksmi further had avoidance of social situations due to this problem. In exploring her reaction she was able to recognize that her mind found many sights, smells, and events repulsive. Visual images of taking care of her cat's litter box would bring her nausea and gagging at just the thought. Indeed, these are some pretty strong thoughts, feelings, and images!

Common to all the mood disorders is my favorite mood disorder word: florid. Florid thoughts are fully developed, and more; they are a whole "scene." Florid thoughts might be abundant, excessive, vivid, grandiose, dramatic, certainly not incomplete and certainly not dull—the bouquet of the thought world.

Imagine, if you will, having thoughts that are so abundant and complete that it is like a bouquet of flowers. Now, if it is a nice bunch of mixed flowers that would be a pleasant scene, perhaps one for a still painting. But if it is a giant bunch of lilacs in a small stuffy room, it could be pretty pungent. And, if it were a 30-day-old bunch of roses from a lover who had left you, it could look pretty dingy and have lots of emotions of pain associated.

That's how life is with florid thoughts

Despite medical treatment, a degree of florid thoughts continues. Florid thoughts are related to the CI (Creative Imaginative) ability of the brain that seems to be strong in many the mood disorders. The book, *Touched by Fire,* recounts the incredible list of creative persons who have the mood disorders. Although actual research and textbooks do not fully support the creative link to the mood disorders, my therapy experience has been just that bipolar patients just seem to have the creative flair.

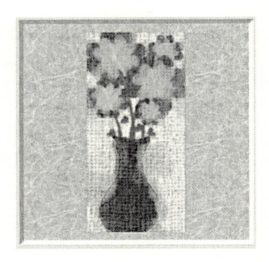

In severe bipolar disorder, it is easy to track periods of creativity and productivity to periods of mania and depression of the great painters and musicians. Unfortunately for them, personally, today's mood stabilizers did not exist then. Hemingway committed suicide, Mozart demonstrated bizarre behavior in public, and the Marquis de Sade wrote books with his own blood. In the mild moods, these patterns are less defined, but florid thoughts and creativity are still present!

Consider these real life situations where florid thoughts are present:

John was having difficulty with extreme sensitivity to smells and touch, which was inhibiting his sex life. He was finding it too "messy" and just could not get over some bad past experiences with "bad smells." He felt this was an insurmountable barrier with his partner, but did not know that florid thinking was to blame.

Bill has ongoing dysphoric (pained, the opposite of euphoric) feelings about some household chores that his wife gives him. This is related to forced chores and depression as a child. On Saturdays, he develops a deep heaviness and feels like he can't lift his arms. He knows this is a bit silly, because his arms could not become heavier on Saturdays. Bill explored florid thoughts, and sought to find some ways to intervene with this strong reaction.

Linda has severe pain, which her doctor has not been able to help her with. She is exploring this as both real pain and florid thoughts.

Jay has strong senses. His ability to taste is very strong. He also states that he can walk into a room and pick up odors. Foods and smells can be extremely pleasurable or incredibly distracting.

The imagination combined with florid thoughts can take fears that are normal to the average person and make them into that flowery bouquet—a giant unmanageable one. Nightmares become images that do not disappear the next day, but become quandaries about life. Odd images in the brain become questions:

- Was I molested?

- Did I see a spacecraft?

- Is someone following me?

- Is there some toxic poison on my skin?

- Are they going to fire me?

- Will I fail at ____?

- Do they hate me?

- Is my nose misshapen?

- Will God send me to hell?

The odd questions can be endless.

Nightmares can occur during the day. These daytime images or flashes can cause a moment of fear as the movie-like scene pans in front of a person.

Jane came into a session and stated that she had an image of a horrible accident on the Interstate and said that in her past she often has had premonitions of accidents. The next week she reported back that no accident had occurred. She took some time to explore her florid thoughts that were being expressed as images during the day, seeming premonitions that caused her panic and disrupted her life. She agreed to stop, breathe, and work on encapsulating or containing these images despite the realistic feelings in them.

My dad, a vault of worldly wisdom, was telling me about a person lost in the woods in central Idaho. An eccentric lady we both knew showed up at the search zone and volunteered to help. She said that she could help because by using her ability to "smell death" she could tell where the lost person is. Here is a person in touch with florid thoughts and, whether or not she actually could do this, something florid or manic is happening to her.

So, for the "florid person," life is vividly good, vividly bad, or vividly dull. We certainly understand how something could be a party, exciting, and stimulating. But how can life be vividly dull? Many soft bipolars experience depressed states where their main symptoms being where there are very strong mental reactions. Boredom, free time, and minor struggles can be vividly difficult.

Many mild moods describe the dull and depressed phases as a "pained" phase wherein there is actual pain and discomfort. Rather than euphoric, there is the actual opposite, dysphoria. The person is not without thoughts or feelings, they are sensing actual pain.

Sometimes, they feel agitated, unsettled, and uncertain. Certainly, this is a very uncomfortable place to be. For some, there is the heaviness of body and mind. For others, there is complete hopelessness and despair. For the dysthymics, there is irritation, inability to handle stimulation, and need to withdraw. Still, depression is pain. This is why there is a tendency to:

- Pull away from others, hide.

- Escape responsibility.

- Seek any escape (drink, overeat, give up, sabotage anything, act out, cut oneself).

- Entertain hopeless, panicked, or suicidal thoughts.

- Desire to leave this pained world: suicide (Soft bipolars need to be educated on this pain and how to intervene.)

Florid thoughts may lead patients to their doctor's office or to the health food store in search of answers. While some mood disorder sufferers have concerns for illness that is not there (hypochondriasis), others have actual small illnesses that are made more troubling due to the florid. Simply put, the physical symptoms are real, and the floridness exaggerates it.

Trauma

When the mild moods are confronted with a situation where the CI mind does its job, they can get into trouble. In fact, this CI mind never forgets, and the person can be traumatized by events that do not traumatize the average person.

A childhood sleepover becomes a lifetime memory of fear and failure. Fear of the dark or the bogey man goes on into adulthood, causing a married woman to not feel safe in her home at night, keeping this secret from her husband for years.

A horror movie seen as a teenager continues to linger in a mind for years as images of a gory scene pop up often as though the person had post traumatic stress disorder.

Scenes of tragic accidents from local news programs create such horrific fear that a person, who did not have agoraphobia (fear of being away from a safe place or person), eventually develops it, and will not leave their small neighborhood.

All too often, strong fearful images of illness and death keep people from entering hospitals or going to funerals.

Other troubling thoughts can include:

- fearing one's mental health ("I will really go crazy")

- Feeling a relationship will not work out

- feeling you have failed

- Extreme fear of being separated from others

- paranoia of others or what they must be thinking

- pervading sense of doom

- just about any thought that is entrenched in your mind and has been around a long time, often going back to childhood

Kathleen was told to save her pennies when she was a child. To this day she fears running out of money, despite many years of solid paychecks.

Time lock

Mild moods report that they get locked in time, usually the here and now. This is not some existential "I am here in the moment" joyous feeling. Instead, there is the experience of being stuck or looping in some current thought or emotion. It is like quicksand, a bog, cement, and a trap.

For mild moods, this can happen fast. In fact, it can happen in an instant. It is both biological and psychological, this focused fixated locking in the now. The past is forgotten. Hope for the future is forgotten.

Arjun was having a tough time accepting and adjusting to taking a mood stabilizer for the first time, being diagnosed recently as bipolar 2. An A+ student at the local university, he reported he had just got all Cs. His life and future were over, he stated, in session. He was in total despair. He felt all he had lived for was lost in this semester, where some medication trials had disrupted his ability to function

Arjun would eventually get over it, and could even have the university assist with some repair of the grades because bipolar disorder is a disability. But, one would be hard pressed to talk him out of his current pain.

In time lock, the IC mind takes the current situation and creatively blows it out of proportion. You can see how panic and fear can arise so quickly for the mood disorders. In a time lock, it is even hard to get them to stop and take a deep breath, because there is a feeling of terror: the world is about to end.

Certainly, the motto given to kids at crosswalks is good advice here: stop, look, and listen! Those who are beginning time lock patterns may be able to identify the pattern and how it occurs and intervene. After identifying typical patterns, one could keep a reminder around, such as a checklist kept in a wallet or purse. One would want to review this often. Time lock can sneak up pretty fast.

Many have perpetual time lock. Others are more entrenched in bad patterns. They may not be aware when they lock up, but some give themselves "permission" to have a time lock, like throwing a little fit. We all do it, and it seems to be somewhat socially acceptable.

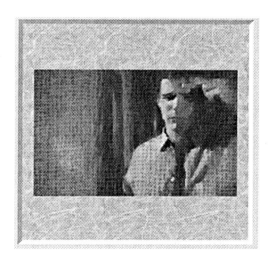

"I always hate Friday traffic, get in an argument, and have to get drunk or take extra Ativan."

"My doctor is never available on Friday afternoons. I get so wound up Saturdays that I throw things at my husband."

"The kids drive me nuts after school."

Time lock can also take two other time variations. Although most get stuck in a current mood, thought, or problem, others don't. For them, there is the sad or traumatic past or the frightening or even hopeful future.

Those living in the past may have periods where they are overly melancholy, live in past hurts, or review past mistakes. Regrets or past traumas can be ever-present in the mind's eye.

Jason always lived with regrets for not going to college. He could not make peace with his reasons for his early choices. His life and conversations often centered on this past.

Olivia, 55, still regrets early marriage to her husband and moving from Maine. During the day, her mind often wanders to sad and melancholy feelings of what she feels she left in wooded Maine. Sadness has become part of her life, and she has to avoid drinking: it triggers her to suicidal thoughts.

Some are always reaching into the future and not able or wanting to be present in the now. There is always some better job, relationship, or life to solve problems. Unfortunately, anxious and depressed planning seldom goes well as it is rooted in fear.

Inner Voice Problems

We all talk to ourselves, whether we will admit this or not. It does not mean we are crazy that we have this inner dialogue going on. Well, it is getting out there a bit if the person answering you back is Elton John or somebody else. Then it is delusional. Otherwise, internal dialogue is pretty normal.

But the mild moods can have several particular inner voice problems. The first is that in any down or depressed phase, there is a mean, cruel, and critical voice that takes over in the head. At that point, there is nothing you can do or say that is right. There are many terms in psychology for this voice—the critical inner parent being one.

This mean, hostile voice is unrelenting, and it is driven by our fears. It will bring up any failure, anything wrong about now, any pimple you might have. It will use just about anything to prove that you, your place in the world, your abilities, and how others will accept you are pretty awful.

Here are critical points about the critical voice:

- It will not stop.

- It is in total error.

Nothing you really do or say will satisfy this voice because it is the voice of depression, anxiety, and pain. What it "says" will always seem to make some sense. It will pick only issues that make the most sense to you and it is going to prod you where you are weakest and most vulnerable.

The inner critic always has something to say that is negative about our worth, our abilities, our life, our relationships, and our safety in the world. What is brought up does hurt and attacks any self-esteem left.

To counter the inner critic, one needs to

- Identify the dark voice.

- Be prepared; it will strike when you least want it.

- Counter this.

- Circumvent this.

- Confront this.

- Stop this.

There are many good books on the Inner Critic, but the one by Hal and Sidra Stone, *Embracing Your Inner Critic, Turning Self-Criticism into a Creative Asset*, is the best.

When you are in a good frame of mind prepare some good reminders to counter the negativity for the negative attacks of depressed states. Keep lists of any type around, stating:

- Who you are: a healthy assessment of yourself usually made during non-depressed times.

- What your life is about, your purpose.

- What your special gifts and talents are.

- What you can do today while depressed to help yourself to move forward.

- Any other helpful information on hope or inspiration you rely on. (There are great life affirmations in A Setback is a Setup for a Comeback, by Willie Jolley.)

- What are your personal, spiritual, or faith resources.

Another voice is the one I call the inner imp. This is the voice that will do whatever behavior with a smirk on its face. It just wants to flaunt convention and rules. This Dennis the Menace, or Pippi Longstocking, character is the little rebel in all of us, but comes out during times of mild or severe mania or boredom:

- To hell with mood charts, books, meds, etc.

- I just sat down with the cake intending to nibble on the frosting and ate the whole thing.

- Why get one blouse when you can get all 10 colors?

- I'm married, but had sex today with two other persons, and without protection.

The inner imp seeks stimulation, fulfillment, rebellions, the now, noise. Lights, cameras, action!

This voice also runs rampant in the manic or mild manic states (hypomania) where a person has less contact with saner inner voices of reason. Those voices are the voices we could call the rational voices. This is the inner wise role, called the inner sage or the observer self. In real mania, experienced by in bipolar 1, those voices of reason are gone altogether. Move over Thelma and Louise. Blast off!

I could always tell when Mild Mood Jay stopped taking his Depakote mood stabilizer. He drove to the office with car windows open and the radio blazing. His vocal volume and jokes quickly resonated throughout the whole building.

Well, we all need to address and be aware of these unconscious voices or inner roles. Or, when you least expect it, they may pop out and take over. If not made aware and worked with "kindly," these voices combine with manicy states leading us into high-risk behavior: drug use, STDs, speeding cars, etc.

If you have further interest in exploring the Inner Critic or Inner Imp, ask your therapist about Jungian "shadow work."

In addition, bipolars have a constant barrage of thoughts from the three other characters:

The inner problem solver—Intrusive thoughts keep running around in the mind. These are small pesky thoughts we sometimes tolerate. This can include a mini-obsession about the traffic or not getting work done.

The inner worrisome self—This character created slightly more anxious thoughts. Often these thoughts center around fear of failure, what people think of us, and how we related to others and the world.

The inner sentinel—This is the creator of giant fears. This character is like a watchtower guard that is way out of control. Fear is generated by any stimuli. The "guard" is frightened by every shadow and noise and goes into fear mode immediately.

I hope to address these three characters in my next book on soft bipolar.

Another way to look at inner voice problems is to identify the out-of-control inner voices. Two particular ones running crazy are the inner problem solver and the inner protector.

The inner problem solver is simply our innate mechanism that seeks to solve problems. Out of control, it starts an endless loop of thinking that is a pest: rumination.

The stronger version, the inner protector, is that role within that seeks to protect us from harm. If it gets too jazzed up, it creates terrifying images and scenarios about situations that may not be truly harmful. We will examine these in my next book, to come out the summer of 2005, *More on Soft Bipolar*.

Obsessive, compulsive and more fear-driven behavior

Obsessive-compulsive disorder (OCD) is the brain disorder where a person has fear and repeated rituals. Remember the movie, As Good As It Gets, where Jack Nicholson's character was washing his hands over and over? That's OCD. Many persons with OCD would like to stop their repeated behavior.

Many bipolar sufferers get transient OCD during severe mixed-state moods, and fearful washing of clothes, fear of counting and taking pills, fear of germs can engulf a life.

Oddly, not all OCD sufferers are also perfectionists. They may be obsessed about cleaning the microwave for germs, but have a fridge full of old and harmful foods.

Obsessive-compulsive personality disorder (OCPD) is often not diagnosed and is, I think, present in many bipolar sufferers. The OCPD person has anxious and perfectionist tendencies. Things must be done right, perfectly, right now. They tend to worry a lot of the time. And, unlike OCD, they would like to do it more and get even better at what they are obsessive and compulsive about.

Craig knows OCPD is a large part of his mood problems. When he gets obsessed about finding the just the correct software for his computer, he will spend hours each day working on this. He can't stop until the project is satisfied, and then, on to another obsession. His wife knows he is obsessive about foods and vitamins, personal hygiene, and order in general.

Those with OCPD are the "control" side of the Soft Bipolars. They do need to lighten up, to go with the flow, and to learn to flex. Otherwise, anxiety can rule. On the other side of the spectrum are those with less need for control. These persons are more impulsive, and due to low impulse control get into the most trouble with drugs, alcohol, risky behavior, outbursts, etc.

The polarized life is like a hot fudge sundae

These core issues—florid thoughts, time lock, voice problems, and self esteem issues—rob joy from life. They also tend to make life more extreme compared to the lives of others.

But it can feel totally normal to you.

Ego and stress collapse—when you fall apart

Because of the extremeness and stress of these thoughts, a secondary problem is created for some. Some persons fall apart under the stress of all of this.

The up and down nature of bipolar mood disorder takes a toll, not just on the quality of life, but also on the physical brain. As stress increases one suffers and emotional collapse called "decompensation."

Decompensation is like Humpty Dumpty. The children's rhyme says that Humpty Dumpty had a great fall. Well, mood disorder sufferers can "fall apart," too. They have periods where they fracture, or emotionally unravel at the seams. This decomposition is like a great robot, all out of juice, that shuts down completely. This shutting down is both emotional and biological.

Mood stabilizers combined with therapy seek to lessen collapses. Holding it together is an important thing to do in life!

If you would like to examine some ways to confront disturbing and frightening thoughts from a fun mythical manner, check out the book, *Mind Monsters,* at www.MoodDisorder.net.

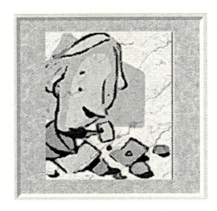

5

Meet the Soft Bipolars: Bipolar 1 and 2

I was glad Jay had finally made it through the first two years of his new marriage. Twice before, he had not made it this far as he divorced at the eighteenth-month point in both relationships.

Jay met Caroline at a very cheery bar and later showered her with all the romantic gifts a person could think of. But after the marriage, losing his personal space quickly stressed him out. He went from being irritable to a mental collapse, where he could not function. He felt the pressures placed on him—and blame. This caused him to give up his routines of golf and time out with the guys. Jay initially did not see that in relationships he collapsed under pressure and had a shift in mood. His emotions went out of control.

Typically, Jay would have been misdiagnosed with many different problems in the counseling office, including being just depressed, being narcissistic, self-centered, stressed and traumatized, (each of which was present to a small degree).

But, Jeff had other "markers"—clues to mood disturbances in his life. In his family, there were suggestions of hidden mood disorders. For him, patterns in relationships and jobs showed that this bright person had patterns in starting and ending relationships based on mood phases. Employment too had this roller coaster effect.

Jeff is typical of the many mild moods: you have to look hard to see that he would fit the diagnostic criteria for two important disorders that would give him access to needed help: bipolar 2 and cyclothymia. These two disorders, in brief, are:

Bipolar 2—This is the "functional" type of Bipolar Disorder, a mood disorder. It is characterized by periods of depression and periods of elevated mood that is not "manically high," called hypomania.

Cyclothymic disorder (Some call this bipolar 3, while others reserve bipolar 3 for those with mood cycles induced by drugs or a depressed child of an alcoholic parent)—Cyclothymic disorder is a very mild form of bipolar disorder characterized by mild mood changes: mild depression and mild excitement. Mood shifts exist, but are related to activating events. The more severe mood disorders have cycling not always triggered by some life event. Here, the depression is just milder. If bipolar 1 is the roller coaster, this is the kiddy ride.

If untreated, about 40 percent of cyclothymics will eventually develop bipolar 1 or 2 ("The Bipolar Spectrum" in *Archives of Medicine, JAMA* and *Archives,* www.archfami.ama-ama-assn.org).

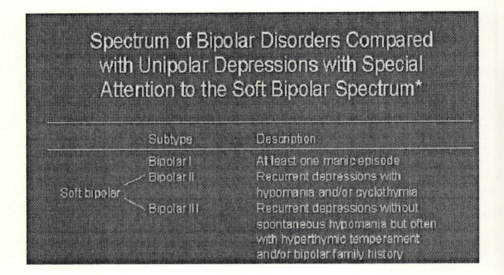

(From *Bipolar II and III: Interface of Temperament and Soft Bipolarity* by Hagop S. Akiskal, MD, at the Second International Conference on Bipolar Disorder) www.wpic.pitt.edu/stanley/2ndbipconf/)

Some would feel that Jeff would not fit the two categories above because there is not enough mood shifting. It is hard to see that his life is bi-phasic, where there is an up and down mood state (hence, we get the term bipolar from having two mood phases, or "poles."

But if we could spend time, day to day, with Jeff, we might be able to see that he, indeed, is experiencing these shifts in mood, but he himself is not aware that it is occurring. One major influence in the work of the field of mood disorders, German neuropsychiatrist Kraepelin, said that many mood disorder patients will not be truly known until you see them on a daily basis.

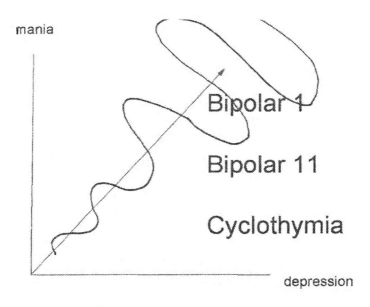

(This is the European view of Cyclothymia)

Now, everybody has moods, and not all moods represent a mood disturbance. Not all mood disturbances are mood disorders. The following behaviors are indicative of persons with normal moods. The average person:

- can read for a block of time and enjoy that

- In a conversation can talk, but also listen

- does not push limits just to stir things up

- completes tasks; can stay on task

- has typical and normal anxieties

- has periods of quietude and calm

- is able to sleep a majority of time

- is able to accept criticism most of time from another person without becoming reactive

- can feel loss, frustration, and confusion for normal periods of time

- can experience a range of emotions and not be overtaken by an emotion for days

- can resolve problems in typical amounts of time, albeit difficult, etc.

In the mild moods, whether we look at bipolar 2 or cyclothymia, we are looking at extremes. The bipolarity, or up and down nature, may be not observable to the common eye, but the vividness or extremeness is there.

"Soft bipolar" refers to a broader definition of the milder mood disorders–those other than bipolar 1. Several different lists of subtypes of the mood disorders have been suggested:

Klerman, 1987

Bipolar 1: mania and depression

Bipolar 2: hypomania and depression

Bipolar 3: cyclothymic disorder

Bipolar 4: hypomania or mania precipitated by antidepressant drugs

Bipolar 5: depressed patients with a family history of Bipolar 1Illness

Bipolar 6: mania without depression (unipolar mania)

Akiskal, 1999

Bipolar 1: full-blown mania

Bipolar 1 ½: depression with protracted hypomania

Bipolar 2: depression with hypomanic episodes

Bipolar 2 ½: cyclothymic disorder

Bipolar 3: hypomania due to antidepressant drugs

Bipolar 3 ½: hypomania and/or depression associated with substance use

Bipolar 4: depression associated with hyperthymic temperament

(Actual journal references and more details are available at www.psychom.net/ depression.central.lieber.html)

For the mild moods, overall symptoms may include symptoms that look to others like separation anxiety, marked irritability, or oversensitivity to emotional or environmental triggers. (Papolos in www.geocities. com/ptypes/Cyclothymicpd.html)

Often, the bipolarity may only be seen when other disorders or life issues are cleared out of the way:

Jane was having panic attacks. After treatment for that, she began to disclose problems with mild mood shifting she had experienced all her life.

Many bipolar 2s show up on my counseling doorstep, referred by a relative or the courts for legal or marital problems. They often have gotten themselves into trouble for gambling, impulsiveness, getting several DUIs, or something else that is a clue to a mood disorder. These are the functional Bipolars. They have jobs and relationships but may secretly struggle to hold it all together.

Mild moods are most likely to:

- change jobs;

- lose focus;

- divorce;

- quit school;

- not meet their potential.

Not all of these characteristics fit all soft bipolar persons. But the comprehensive lists in this book, should help you get the picture. You may want to pick and choose to make your own list.

Symptoms may include, but do not always include, the up or hypomanic side:

cheerful

exuberant

optimistic

self-aware

boastful

energetic

versatile

stimulus seeking

short sleeper

irritable

happy

enhanced senses

increased intelligence or creativity

distracted

accelerated thoughts

decreased inhibitions

increased libido

feels good physically

starts projects

excessive

fast.

colorful

flamboyant

social

likes noise and stimulation

does several things at once

negligent driving

increased appetite

others seen in slow motion

spending

poor judgment

itching

greater sensitivity

increased alcohol or tobacco use

feels hot

mild euphoria

excessive writing

approaches delusions, almost paranoid

fault finding

vivid or grandiose imagery

vivid tastes

On the down, depressed side, symptoms and behaviors can, but don't always, include:

gloomy.

humorless

guilt

sluggish

slow, passive

devoted

long sleep

anxiety

panic

self-deprecation

unexplained fears

lethargic

morbid preoccupation

lowered consciousness

lowered output

decreased verbal output

less talk

withdrawal

mental confusion

memory problems

tearfulness

melancholy

self absorbed

ruminative or stuck thoughts

dull

skeptical or paranoid

compulsions

lack of interests

may feel ill or sick

overwhelmed by stimulus

feels cold

vivid dark images

goes to a dark place

indecision

heavy heart, burdened

foggy, feels like a mist

feels heavy, leaden arms or legs

sore, tired

North and South Pole

Some may feel they don't fit this "two pole" up and down, or bi-phasic, category at all. Indeed, there are those who are continually in one mood phase. This includes especially those who are consistently in one phase, like the always-happy hyperthymic or the always-depressed dysthymics. On the Internet are several web sites recounting personal stories of a life of elevated and chipper mood, hyperthymic temperament: http://home.att.net/~s.l.keim/MyStory.html and http://www.biopsychiatry.com/happiness/hyperthymia.html

Included in this missing north and south pole picture might be those who have taken many antidepressants, experience much anxiety, and have a more mixed-up picture. We will cover mixed states in the next chapter. And it can get pretty darn complicated, just as you are a very complicated person, both in your brain and in your temperament.

There are just dozens of variations on this whole picture. A person's mood pattern can be influenced by many factors, including secondary disorders and a person's resilience to problems.

Kim grew up in a stable family with lots of resources and security. While many of his relatives had severe bipolar disorder, it seemed that his own stable environment contributed to his having only a very mild mood disorder.

Margarida was traumatized as a child by parental conflict and verbal abuse. She was never able to fully recover from this. While most persons in her family were only noted to be alcoholics, Margarida still struggles to find mood stabilizing medications and therapy that helps her deal with frequent mental collapses.

Henry was diagnosed as a child with bipolar 2. Later in life he frequently took heroine and methamphetamine. Due to this, he has moved over to a diagnosis of bipolar 1 and is in and out of psychiatric hospitals often.

No two bipolar sufferers are exactly alike.

There are those who feel agitated in either mood state.

There are those who don't feel agitated in these states.

There are those who feel anxiety in either state.

There are those who don't feel anxiety in either state.

There are those who feel a little more "together" in the mood states.

And then there are those who feel less collected, less connected with the world and others.

Contrasting worlds

Lists of contrasting moods and energy states can help us detect when bipolarity occurs. These contrasting word lists should be included in any evaluation for the mood disorders.

Do you have varying periods of:

- sharpened and creative thinking alternating with periods of mental confusion and apathy

- good mood versus times of irritable mood

- loss of interest or pleasure versus elevated and expansive mood

- decreased need for sleep versus too much need for sleep

- shaky self esteem and lack of self confidence versus naïve grandiose overconfidence

- unusual work hours with much done versus periods of down time and recuperation

- more uninhibited people seeking or social good times versus introverted self-absorption

- involvement in pleasurable activities versus restricted involvement in pleasurable actives and guilt over past activities

- optimism or exaggeration of past achievement versus pessimistic attitude toward the future or brooding about past events

- more talkative than usual with laughing, joking, and punning versus less talkative with tearfulness or crying

- financial extravagance versus periods of guilt and self punishment.

- more sexual or impulsive versus over-constraint or held-back.

- shopping, spending, and doing versus low activity.

- feeling in slow motion versus feeling in fast motion.

- feeling serious or morbid versus happy.

- feeling like your body is heavy versus your feel light or energetic.

(Adapted from "Cyclothymic Personality Disorder" in www.geocities.com/ptypes/Cyclothymicpd.html)

Some don't like the "contrasting worlds" idea

Many soft bipolars, when they stop and think about it, can see that they function in different mood states. Perhaps fifty percent have awareness this is currently happening, but many can see the mood change only in retrospect.

Soft bipolar is always rapid cycling. Rapid cycling refers to mood swings that are shorter in duration that bipolar 1. Often, bipolar 1s have mood swings that are many months or years. Soft bipolars have more rapid mood cycling of several times per year. Some may have mood shifts during a week, a day, or even hours.

Sue was discussing with me in therapy a recent conflict with her boyfriend. Interspersed were comments and moods about the incredibly fantastic aspects that also existed in the relationship. As she moved from the good to the bad stuff, her mood switched. She noted that during the mood shifts she went from feeling euphoric and elated about the relationship, to feeling depressed and hopeless. Sue was rapid cycling with fast changing moods that were distinctly observable.

Cole mentioned in a bipolar treatment class that he was cycling about every minute. This had followed a period of depression and happy hypomania. Cole had stopped taking his anti-manic medication and was actually moving into a mild mania. While he felt he was rapid cycling, the pattern actually indicated he was feeling the rapid highs and lows of mild mania, despite feeling depressed from one moment to the next euphoric feeling

Some people who feel an ultra rapid cycle are actually in hypomanic or manic states, as erratic moods accompany these. Mixed mood states also are erratic.

Up Mood State

Rapid Erratic Cycling but
is actually hypomanic or manic

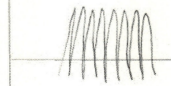

a 24-hour period or even just an hour

Down Mood State

Up Mood State

Rapid Cycling

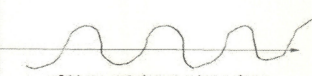

a 24-hour period or even just an hour

Down Mood State

Some Soft Bipolars don't fully accept the idea of full mood shifts in terms of an up and down phase. Rather, they see themselves as always creating a constant barrage of vivid thoughts and emotions, and it really does not matter whether it is anger or joy; it is just part of the flowing torrent in their mind.

These people see their disorder as not truly Bipolar, or bi-phasic, but an uncontrolled perpetual flow of thought and emotion. Biological ideas on the lessened mood/emotion/thought control in the Bipolar person's brain may support this: the frontal lobes of the brain do not as actively mediating thoughts and mood as is done in other persons' brains. Indeed, and unfortunately, in autopsies, Bipolar sufferers are noted to have less of this frontal lobe matter in their brain, the part that regulates the flow of ideas and brings about rational thinking.

Some persons note both: notable mood shifts with the perpetual barrage of shifting mini moods. I find that many patient websites support this continual flow idea for Soft Bipolar as people describe their own personal experience. Perhaps in the future some types of Soft Bipolar may be called something like "thought and mood dysregulation disorder".

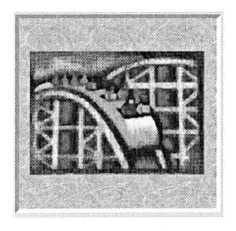

6

Four mood disorder types

There are common factors of the mild moods, especially the florid thoughts, which most have, including florid depression or florid happiness. But there are distinct subtypes of mild moods. If you put a bunch of them in a room, they might have a hard time relating because it would be such a distinct mix of the bubbly, the withdrawn, and the anxious.

Some characteristics of soft bipolars go away with treatment. There are still subtypes of these soft bipolars. There are also characteristics of people that do not go away; these would be called soft bipolar temperament types. We are going to jumble them a bit together in this chapter, and you see what goes away with treatment. What is leftover would be your ongoing soft bipolar temperament type. Medication for treatment is absolutely essential, but individuals that are not warned about ongoing temperament issues are caught off guard when temperament issues flare.

Temperament typing in mental health is not that common these days. Seldom do I come across another practitioner who uses the Myers-Briggs Type Indicator or other temperament tests, which seem to have wide acceptance in the area of business training and development.

But lo and behold, in the field of mood disorders, temperament type is a valid characteristic—as valid as saying the shirt is blue. While people have brain disorders, such as panic or common depression, temperament is not seen as a vital factor to be addressed. But with mood disorders, it is important to both proper diagnosis and treatment of the person. (If you enjoy temperament typing, check out this contemporary view of Mr. Spock and Luke Skywalker in the book *People Patterns: A Modern Guide to the Four Temperaments,* by Stephen Montgomery, Ph.D.).

Ancient temperament typing

Temperament typing goes back thousands of years. Originating with Hippocrates, the Greek physician (c. 460–377 BC), the "four ancient temperaments" of

Greece described suspected fluids coursing though a person's body that created temperament:

- sanguine–happy and social

- choleric–serious, irritable, and hard working, obsessive and compulsive

- melancholy–serious thinking, gloomy

- phlegmatic–easy going, carefree

In the field of mood disorders, there have been studies to document subtypes of temperaments or personalities as:

- cyclothymic temperament (a milder form of cyclothymia, sort of like "traits of cyclothymia) cycling mood, mild shifts

- depressive

- irritable

- hyperthymic

(Akiskal, HS, *Journal of Affective Disorders,* 1998, October, Issue 51, 07-19)

I would like to look at four mood disorder temperament types in this chapter:

- soft bipolar type 1–the mini-roller coaster of cyclothymic temperament

- soft bipolar type 2–born to be happy–the hyperthymics

- soft bipolar type 3–depressed or irritable

- soft bipolar type 4–mixed state–the pain of agitation, tired, and wired all at the same time

Soft bipolar mood type 1

The mini-roller coaster of cyclothymic temperament

These persons may have a regular pattern of mood cycling, but mood disturbance may also follow patterns of stress, work, and the day of the week. These are the mild moods that are seen as bi-phasic: bubbly in one situation, down and depressed in another.

Here are some possible variations of this mini-mood roller coaster. Some have a somewhat predictable or regular pattern, but some shifts are precipitated by stressful events, such as life crisis (fired from job, graduate from college, get married, medical problems, etc.)

Which is it: cyclothymia (soft bipolar) or cyclothymic temperament? Cyclothymia is the milder form of Bipolar 2, a biological disorder. But the even milder form is cyclothymic temperament. Some individuals have cyclothymic temperament without having bipolar disorder. And, some bipolars have ongoing cyclothymic temperament. In our examples here, we are looking at persons with soft bipolar that even when treated with medication have ongoing mild mood cycles from cyclothymic temperament.

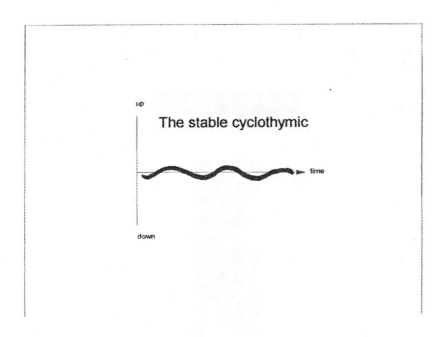

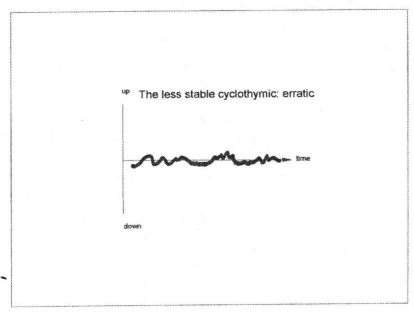

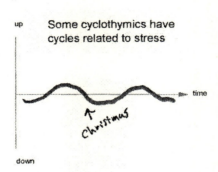

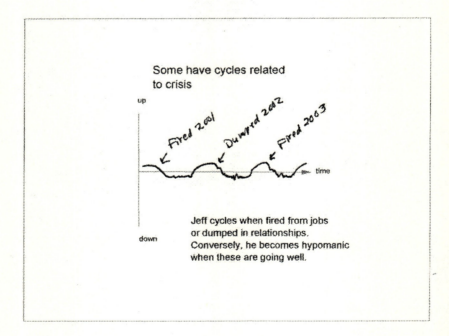

Soft bipolar mood type 2

Born to be happy—the hyperthymics

These are the people born to be happy. These people have all the classic positive benefits of the hypomanic traits, including being exuberant, extroverted, and stimulus seeking. They call themselves the life of the party, and indeed, when they show up, the party begins.

Let's add a few descriptors to our prior "up" list that might characterize the hyperthymics:

talkative

may be the life of the party but may scare others off

looks for fun and games

blustery

humorous, Likes dating and comedy

poor planners

gets angry easily

exaggerates

elaborates

controlled by the present

lives in the present

charms others

would rather talk than _____

starts flashy, finishes poorly

wastes time talking

undisciplined

decides by feelings

volunteers for jobs, but gets distracted

looks great on surface, but may be shallow

high ideals, but gives up

priorities out of order

makes things fun, but chaotic

doesn't listen to whole story

is liked by others, but misses responsibilities

doesn't hold grudges, but interrupts

fickle

repeats

refreshing

haphazard

messy

scattered

show-off

unpredictable

dominates

imprudent planning

uninhibited

loses money, resources

(Adapted from www.longevitywatch.com/temperaments.htm, and Akiskal 1992 at www.wpic.pitt.edu/stanley.2ndbipofconf/)

I attach the word "euthymic" here. There are those who report that they never have a down moment. Euthymic refers to always being in normal mood state. But the euthymic/hyperthymic has one state—up. Most people who like to call themselves hyperthymics are truly bi-phasic bipolar 2s who are not aware of short periods of depression, and their social and gregarious nature puts them at great risk. Happy hour at the bar or party drug use will be the catastrophic event that will open up bipolar 1 mood disorder. They are at risk for switching to a more serious disorder as something triggers or "activates" bipolar 1 to open up and bloom.

Now, I don't want to rain on anyone's parade, and a hyperthymic always interprets it such. But, the hyperthymic/euthymic is in trouble when:

- There are indications of bipolar mood disorder in their family.

- They may be at risk for developing bipolar mood disorder 1.

- They may be covering up or not understanding that there are actually depressive periods, which they just see as down time, fatigue time, sick time.

- They are actually sometimes experiencing mania.

- They are getting into risky behavior and situations, such as gambling sprees, over-spending, sex addictions, speeding, etc.

Hyperthymics just seem to attract a lot of luck in finding jobs and love. To be bubbly and to be "out there" gets you networked, observed, and liked really fast. While some of my patients may work on trying to get a date for years, a hyperthymic will only have to give it minutes. Hyperthymics just seem to roll in job offers, ideas, etc. They don't need to read their astrology; it just rolls out for them.

But, as a disorder, there are real downsides as listed above. When I know a hyperthymic is going to start dating, I always have my "safe sex" talk with them because hyperthymics show poorer judgment. While not usually ending up with catastrophic sexually transmitted diseases such as AIDS, they often come back to another session and report they got herpes simplex virus. Perhaps they asked their partner some safe sex questions, maybe about AIDS, but have not been fully observant of sores.

For extreme hyperthymics,

- sociability can become periods of irresponsibility;

- starting projects can be too expansive;

- ideas can flow too freely;

- others can be convinced to the point of being conned.

- humor can be crude;

- social norms can be exceeded;

- boundaries can be overstepped.

Hyperthymics can get wound up, overly optimistic, lose track of things or money, have interests that are too broad, and be scattered.

In marriages, while most are not promiscuous, their spouses for some "mysterious" reason do not trust them. While not bad intentioned, hyperthymic can get stuck at the store or bar for hours and forget others who may want or need them. While they may not plan an affair, they may just "accidentally" get into one because their personal boundaries are so open.

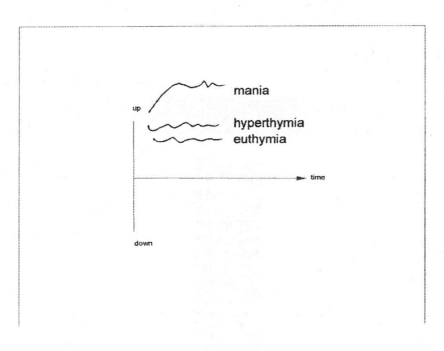

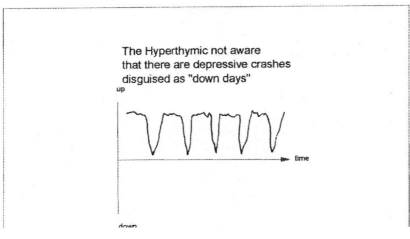

The hyperthymics are often the emotional ones. But when is life, behavior, or emotion too intense? Some H/Es report that emotion can escalate to the point that it can become unbearable and greatly troubling. They then become overwhelmed with human emotions; the volume gets turned too high.

Greta often brings up the fear of her mother's death in session. Although her mother is doing just fine, Greta feels that she would not be able to handle not the death, but her profound emotions she would experience at that time. Prior experiences with strong emotions have proven that she becomes almost incapacitated with the vividness of emotions. Fortunately for Greta, this fear of being overwhelmed keeps this person on track with taking her mood stabilizing medication and attending a mood disorder treatment class, monthly.

David, a hyperthymic, wanted to show me his scars in the first session. He said he was a male version of Pippi Longstocking, which he often read to his daughters. He was that odd, magical person, and had scars from daggers, bullets, sticks, and other things to prove it all. He was proud of this. Unfortunately, David, the son of two alcoholics, was having increased panic attacks and had failed prior antidepressant treatment and therapy for those. He agreed to try a mood stabilizer for the panic only if it would not interfere with his personality. In treatment, he also looks at ways to prevent the drinking problems of his parents.

Shana was in for counseling because her husband was tired of paying for high-risk insurance. Shana had many speeding tickets, putting her in a high-risk category. Each time Shana was arrested, it followed a time when she had stopped taking her mood stabilizer. She was thought by the police to be intoxicated because of her jocular mood. Because of this, each speeding ticket also had complicated arrest issues and legal fees that the typical person would not have. Shana was having a hard time admitting that it was at this point that her jovial mood was out of control, and in fact was possibly moving to a more serious mood disorder.

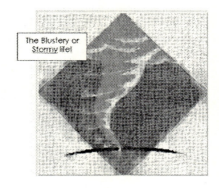

The Blustery or Stormy life!

Soft Bipolar Type 3

Depressed or irritable

The depressed and irritables have a hard time getting appropriately diagnosed and then validated for their soft bipolar. They also may suffer ongoing depression despite medication. This can lead to personal blame and then backing out of treatment altogether. It is likely that these folks have had depression since childhood. They are often part of a group that has suffered from childhood and now the depression and subsequent coping lifestyle may just seem normal. Because of this, they may not even seek treatment.

They come from several possible situations:

• Children of alcoholics, possibly a quiet child who was also neglected.

• Children from quiet, yet mildly depressed, families, for two or more generations. They may whisper a bit, their parents may have been responsible persons, but whisper, too.

• Quiet child with mild depression in childhood, not a troublemaker.

When a person comes from one of these situations, the interpretation is again that to be depressed is normal. Who would think that the shy child in the back of the grade-school classroom is experiencing depression?

It is estimated that one-fourth of all persons depressed are mood disorder depressed. That means that 25 percent of all persons who will start on regular antidepressants instead of mood stabilizers may be heading for trouble.

The mild mood type 3s are like Milne's character Eeyore in the *Winnie the Pooh* books. Eeyore is the gloomy, serious, thoughtful character. He stands in a mud puddle and has a rain cloud over him. His tail falls off. But he certainly brings some needed seriousness to that sanguine Tigger, who just wants to bounce all over the place!

The mild mood depressed are often "functionally depressed." That is, they live with mild depression, think it is normal, and have an adaptive lifestyle that works around it. They still can hold down jobs and some relationships.

Juanita is a mild mood depressed who has her work and home life down to many safe routines. Evenings, her children spend many hours alone doing their homework while she unwinds with large romance novels. Life percolates along pretty safely in this small jar, but if her family tries to interface with her, or there is a change at work, she gets out of control.

Recently, training days at work messed up several routines causing a deeper depression that took several weeks to move out of. It was difficult to explain to Juanita that she has mild depression and then occasionally more serious periods of depression. This has just felt like her normal life to her.

She moved out of her total depression and more mood swings became evident. She saw "the light of day" as she had more times of not being depressed. This brought about some psychic dilemmas as she had based her life on being depressed and did not know how to live life out of the former "coma."

Now, Juanita is involved with more personal interests and is taking her family to more social events that she avoided before.

There might be several different depressed types:

- those who are quiet, calm

- those who are more agitated, with more nervousness

- those with more anxiety, such as panic or social phobias

- those with more irritability

- those with more severe depressive periods or foggy states

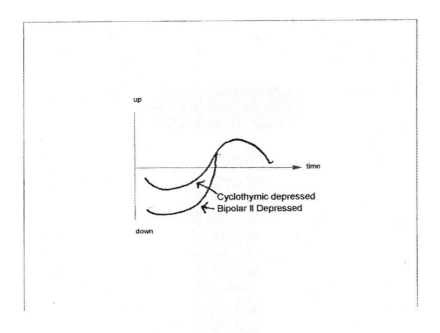

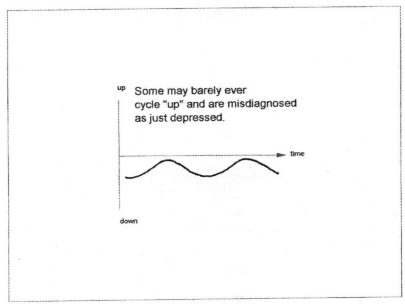

(again, the European view of Cyclothymia)

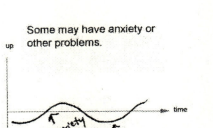

Some may have anxiety or other problems.

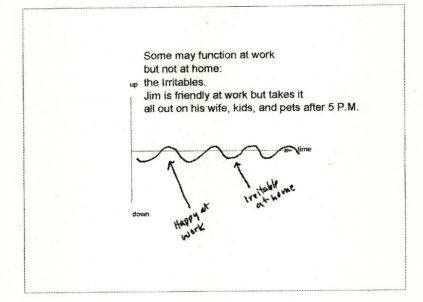

Some may function at work but not at home: the Irritables.
Jim is friendly at work but takes it all out on his wife, kids, and pets after 5 P.M.

She saw a psychiatrist and started taking a mood stabilizer. Over time, I have noticed these types of Depresseds:

- those who feel depression is normal and don't want a change

- those who have depression with various forms of anxiety: generalized anxiety, panic, social phobias, fear of air travel, severe fear of public speaking, social phobia, agoraphobia, odd and unusual phobias

- those with some form of attention deficit disorder

- those with some pain disorders such as chronic fatigue and other problems. (These are called somatic disorder depresseds. Somatic depresseds get various true illnesses that are not made up in the mind. It is not sure why this happens, but these are not fictional, which would be psychosomatic illnesses. These are a very serious problem of the soft bipolar depressed).

Cyclothymic Depresseds note some, but not all, of these characteristics:

- unfounded low self esteem

- unfounded anxiety or paranoia regarding others or one's safety (home, fear of flying, etc.)

- general concentration problems (may have hidden attention or learning problems, too)

- cycling periods of more serious concentration problems

- energy problems

- sleep problems

In addition to the depressed symptoms listed in the prior chapter, depresseds sometimes state they feel physically:

- awkward

- have reduced peripheral vision

- are not athletic

- are slower than others

- are different than others physically

- are more fragile physically than others

- worry about their health

- can't relate to comments of others about robustness of health or the "fire in the belly" drive of others

- are not physically driven

- worry they are sloth-like and slow

- are therefore prone to more injuries than others

- bruise more easily

- are less resilient physically

- recovery less readily from exercise or vacations

- fatigue quickly

    Some may comment that they feel:

- stuck

- painfully bored, while others feel okay

- responsible

- burdened

- slow

- overwhelmed

If treated earlier, rather than later, people like Juanita tend to have more gains in life. That is, they get a few successes in socializing and it tends to accumulate. Life can be lived a bit "larger."

Some cyclothymic depressed may disguise themselves pretty darn well–you'd never know it:

- the quiet neighbor next door

- the teen who writes dark gothic poetry but gets "A"s on it

- the good employee who never participates in any company functions

- the aunt who has two bipolar disorder brothers, but her only characteristic is that she whispers

I also think that the irritables fit into this category with the whisperers and the responsibles. Generally, they don't know that they are irritable; they are experiencing something else in their mind, such as pain or frustration. But for a small child, who has grown up with an irritated parent, the irritability is seen as a pretty caustic thing and always is a negative influence on the course of one small life.

Many irritated bipolar 2s have a pattern of holding mood together during the day (work), but unleashing it all on family (kids and dog) at night.

7

Soft bipolar type 4: mixed-state and anxiety disorders–the pain of agitation, tired and wired all at the same time

In this chapter we will look at the anxious soft bipolar type as well as some of the other anxiety problems of all types of soft bipolar.

Wouldn't it be nice if everybody would just fit into some nice little category, a box, so to speak? But there are those who are called mixed-states and then those who have other disorders that we will address in this chapter.

The mixed-up ones, mixed-states, have both symptoms of being up and down at the same time. It is like a hot fudge sundae, hot and cold. That's what this is; symptoms of the manic or hypomanic state exist along with depressive symptoms.

Maybe you have had to stay up to study for some college exam or take a cross-country trip using NoDoze. That is similar. Tired and wired at the same time. Now, amplify that by 10. Mixed-states can include:

- agitation

- feeling disorganized

- irritation

- worry

- feeling something is going to happen

- feeling tired, but may need to pace

- apprehension

- dysphoria, not feeling good, which is just the opposite of a feeling of euphoria, and this can be pretty bad for the mixed-states, including going on for weeks or years

- inability to sleep, tired during the day

- depressed mood

- rapid thoughts

- lack of flexibility

- may persevere on some issue because of internal anxiety and fear; can't get off a topic

- can't wait

- intense responses to any perceived or biological stressor

- rigid responses or needs

- oppositional

- carb or fat craving

- distractible; seems like has attention deficit hyperactive disorder

- separation anxiety

- may be more prone to impulsive or addictive behaviors during this time.

- edgy

- may seem bothersome or irritate spouse or relatives

- may seem like has obsessive-compulsive personality

Formerly, mixed states of moods were thought to be just transitional states for those persons moving from one mood state to another. One felt these when moving from up to down or vice versa. But, there are persons who have constant mixed states, and may just be prone to it because of other brain, temperament, or life features. It is more common these days due to these villains: the SSRI antidepressants and illicit drugs that cause mixed-state bipolar—and there are thousands if not hundreds of thousands of you all these days. (More on this SSRI induced problem, called "bipolar kindling," is presented in the last chapter.)

Three types of mixed states are described:

- the depressed or anxious hypomanic.

- those with agitated depression.

- the depressed with flights of ideas (rapid thoughts).

(Akiskal in www.wpic.pitt.edu/stanlye/2ndbipconf/pptW40413/sld005.htm)

Just like the Hyperthymics, the Mixed-States are in a vulnerable frame of mind when this is happening. They are vulnerable to all sorts of chaos, from being distracted and getting into a car wreck, to drinking too much booze to calm their nerves (it is known for the mood disorders, 60 percent will have problems with substance abuse some time in their lifetimes [www.mmaoonline.net/Protected/99MNMED/9910/Clayton.html]).

The mixed-states have it a bit tougher than those with stable cycles of mood do. They are more prone to:

- take a longer time to recover;

- have a poorer overall prognosis;

- have more suicidal thoughts;

- have more variations in sexual energy;

- have more ongoing anxiety and insomnia.

The mixed-states will be those soft bipolars who will need a closer and more long-term relationship with both their doctor and therapist. It is also possible that they will be the most likely soft bipolar to be diagnosed and treated for a secondary disorder or needing specific medication and therapy interventions.

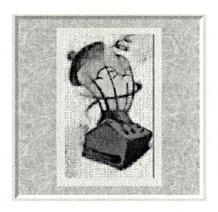

Secondary problems common to mood disorders

As if it is not hard enough having just one disorder, the mood disorders often have more than one psychiatric disorder. This is very, very odd, and very, very unfair in life. The incidence of secondary disorders among bipolar patients is:

- social phobias, 45 percent.

- body dysmorphophobia (the concern that some part of the body is distorted and becoming obsessed about that), 42 percent.

- obsessive-compulsive disorder, 42 percent.

- panic and agoraphobia (the fear of being away from a safe place or person), 64 percent.

- post traumatic stress disorder, 40 percent.

(For a complete listing and description, see www.psycheducation.org/depression/ Anxiety.htm)

Because these disorders are so prevalent in the mood disorders, patients are often misdiagnosed.

Blake has obsessive-compulsive behavior that seems pretty classic. He often is stuck in the boys' bathroom at school and the counselors cannot intervene in his hand washing ritual. At home, Blake lays catatonic on his bed ruminating over his fear of germs and other things.

Although Blake has tried mega doses of anti-obsessional medications, combined with cognitive behavioral therapy, none of these helped. Fortunately, the sixth psychiatrist diagnosed Blake historically as bipolar 2 with SSRI induced cycling. He took him off all anti-obsessional antidepressants, and started mood stabilizers.

One year into treatment, his parents are still skeptical about the long-term help the regimen is supposed to give, but are glad that Blake has avoided residential psychiatric care. The only family history clue to the disorder was others' eccentric behavior. Blake, himself, was noted to be an eccentric child from birth. But, the family and the family's church have a culture of acceptance of this behavior, so it was seen as quite normal.

While a person can have secondary psychiatric disorders, the mood disorders can create disorders, also. For some, this is a transient disorder and for others, the symptoms stick around. Often, there is:

- panic disorder

- obsessive-compulsive disorder, OCD (repetitive behavior tries to stop some ludicrous fear, most common being lengthy hand washing, rereading things, retouching or re-tapping something)

- social phobia and agoraphobia

- general anxiety

We are not sure in all cases, but it there is evidence that these disorders cycle in intensity with the bipolar disorder. And there are specialists who suggest treating the mood disorder because the anxiety symptoms may go away. http://www.psycheductaion.org/depression/Anxiety.htm).

There are other concerns typical of many persons, which are beyond the scope of this book, such as two important topics that are also very common to the mood disorder sufferers: impulsive eating, dieting, (not necessarily the more serious eating disorders) and attention and concentration issues.

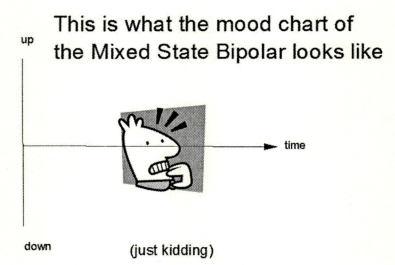

This is what the mood chart of the Mixed State Bipolar looks like

up

time

down   (just kidding)

8

What is bipolar therapy?

Medication and therapy

I always tell patients, mood stabilizers are your lifelines. How, then, does counseling or therapy fit into the picture? The mild moods seldom have inpatient psychiatric stays, but they do sometimes go to emergency rooms or call 9-1-1 when they have anxiety or panic attacks. The soft bipolars are the "walking wounded" of the psychiatric world.

Psychiatrists have less and less time these days to provide information and actual counseling, and the services of licensed therapists are necessary. Some large cities have structured outpatient programs such as my Boise Bipolar Center, which offers individual therapy, as well as patient and family classes.

"Bipolar patients receiving cognitive therapy in addition to medication had significantly fewer bipolar episodes, days ill in an episode, and number of hospital admissions, as well as significantly higher social functioning. There was significantly less fluctuation in manic symptoms among those receiving cognitive therapy, and they also coped better with manic symptoms when they did occur. The findings support the conclusion that cognitive therapy specifically designed for relapse prevention in bipolar illness is useful.

"These findings by Dr. Lam supplement a rapidly growing literature database indicating that a variety of psychotherapeutic strategies (ranging from individual educational work to cognitive-behavioral approaches to family systems psychotherapy) are significantly more effective on a variety of therapeutic outcomes than a control group or treatment as usual. It is no longer a hypothetical construct or presumed supposition, but proven set of findings that patients with bipolar illness should receive appropriately targeted psychotherapy in addition to pharmacotherapies. Significant effects of psychotherapy have also been demonstrated in unipolar affective disorders and a range of anxiety disorders, and therefore these new data in bipolar illness are greatly welcome and help support the contentions that these modalities should be a standard part of Bipolar illness treatment." (from *Bipolar Network News*, Summer, 2003)

And,

"The most comprehensive and advantageous treatment for bipolar illness should involve medication treatment combined with psychotherapy. While bipolar illness is a medical disorder, it is expressed through one's thoughts, mood, social interaction, physical well-being, behavior, and sense of self. Medication treatment is critical, and addresses the severity of the illness, but those living with bipolar illness need the skills and awareness to both make sense of their illness and to develop proactive and reactive approaches to minimize the impact of the illness.

"Psychotherapy offers those with bipolar illness of the illness and issues related to normal living. Treatment that is based on an open and trusting therapeutic relationship can help an individual with bipolar illness distinguish between the debilitating aspect of severe depression and natural experiences of sadness and depressions. Similarly, psychotherapy offers an understanding of the differences between healthy optimism and the boundless unrealistic optimism associated with severe mania.

"Psychotherapy involves an exploration of patterns—in one's thoughts, moods, and behavior. Through such exploration, patients can learn to recognize how daily life events affect them. Similarly, they can learn skills to cope with life's challenges better."

"Another function of psychotherapy is to help patients understand the meaning they assign to their illness and how that influences their response to it. Psychotherapy can play a tremendous role by helping influence how a patient responds to living with Bipolar 1llness." (from *New Hope for People with Bipolar Disorder* by Jan Fawcett, MD. 2000.

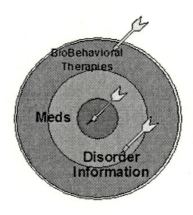

Core targeting in treatment

People need information. The most core treatment is called psychoeducation. The interpretation of bipolar moods and thoughts must come from the basis: "your brain has a disorder and is producing these outlandish moods and thoughts."

Then, people want and need other concrete information. They want to understand the mood disorders, treatment, and the chronic nature of the illness. Then, they want to know what they can do to help their treatment.

Due to the wonderful, evolving nature of this field, I often keep Internet resource files in my waiting room, ask patients to give my copies of anything new they come across on the Net about research or new books, and post new information on a bulletin board in the building. If they are just starting out, I ask them to look up their mild mood type in the Google search engine every few months and see what is new for them to find out.

What doesn't work?

Certainly, the wrong meds and shaky diagnoses hurt and delay treatment. Sometimes, therapists who are well meaning and supportive tend not to exacerbate the illness with bland therapy and still have been helpful assisting undiagnosed patients with life events and crises.

On the other hand, other treatment specialists who give various wrong diagnoses or give advice that exacerbates the illness certainly do not help.

In general, therapies that have been used successfully for mood disorders have included:

CBT: cognitive-behavioral therapy—You can intervene with bad thinking and behaviors, which contribute to mood cycling. There are dozens of books on this as this field has mushroomed for 40 years. If you are not familiar with this and would like to have a simple workbook, just type the above words into the web site at Amazon.com or BarnesandNoble.com, and voila. Your therapist should have readily available handouts and worksheets for you on CBT.

On the down side, if used just formulaically or as stifling homework, some individuals will self-sabotage the work.

IPSRT: interpersonal and social rhythm therapy—If one stabilizes interpersonal issues, cutting out conflict problems, and if one stabilizes life's routines (food, sleep, work, etc.), the medications will work and there will be less cycling. There are still some questions as to whether the patient is most helped by structuring their life or by being brought into a more structured treatment environment with professionals, but it does work.

IPSRT seeks to get individuals back on track with personal habits quickly. Many bipolar specialists feel that the single most important contribution to limiting mood cycling is getting regular sleep. IPSRT leads individuals toward quality sleep habits: no longer can sitting in front of the computer to 3 a.m. be accepted. Getting ready for bed, keeping track of the clock, and doing calming activities such as reading are a part of developing this sleep hygiene.

On the downside, some bipolars resist all the structure IPSRT sets up and are not willing to give up late nights, spontaneity, and sense of freedom. Collaboration in treatment planning is essential. Many Bipolar ls may have some structures imposed on them, such as a frequent violator being required to not work two jobs so that sleep can occur.

Debriefing and insight therapy—Any counseling that helps the mild mood to understand and debrief (you talk about and "release" traumatic emotional content) life events will aid coping.

More and more, counseling includes increased debriefing of life events as we have seen that trauma victims make rapid headway from traumatic events as they recount and process what occurred to them in a counseling setting. For this reason, the Red Cross enlists an "army" of debriefers who go to emergency sites to debrief victims of accidents, floods, etc.

Supportive and problem solving therapies

DBT: dialectical-behavioral therapy—This therapy was developed to assist persons with borderline personality disorder who have special needs. While some bipolar suffers have some traits of borderline personality disorder, DBT is useful for both disorders. I think DBT will be the therapy of choice in the future for all mood disorders, including soft bipolar. Just for your information, borderline personality sufferers are noted for:

- emotional collapses where they rapidly "fall apart at the seems," clinically called "decompensation."

- frequent embroilment in interpersonal conflict with a loved one, obsessed about some aspect of that relationship.

- intense and gripping fears that are out of touch with reality, but seem real (These fears and other dramas can overtake life.)

DBT teaches the patient what these issues are, contracts with the patient regarding the issues, and then, when the issues arise, seeks to manage them.

DBT uses several helpful interventions to accomplish the goal of "holding it together" and staying on course:

- Contingency management: Do I have plans to handle what can go wrong (and, with bipolar persons, jobs, medications, and many things can "go wrong")?

- Self-management skills: How can I manage my time, my job, my home, my life, my routines, my kids, and my _____?

- Core mindfulness methods: What do I do to be aware of my life, my feelings, my disorder, my mood states, my issues, etc.?

- Interpersonal skill building: What skills do I rely on to communicate my feelings and discuss problems with others?

- Grieving skills: how do I work through the emotion of grief?

- Reorientation of attention from wrong focus: How can I keep focused on what is important and how do I get off-track and sometimes obsessed on the wrong issues?

- Contain outlandish thoughts and emotions: See them as generated by a disorder and perhaps not valid in life.

- Look at missing social, personal, or work skills (deficits), and seek to provide these.

DBT has been found to have many crossover benefits with all types of counseling and therapy. For an overview of DBT and information on its developer, see http://www.priory.com/dbt.htm.

Other Methods of Therapy

These therapies remain questionable. In bipolar 1s who have psychosis, they may induce psychotic events. With the mild moods, you should ask you psychiatrist for approval of:

- hypnosis

- visual imagery and neuro-linguistic programming (NLP)

- eye-movement desensitization processing (EMDT).

- psychological weekend workshops called "intensives," retreats, fasts

- unusual psycho/spiritual/physical treatment that is not a normal practice for you or your culture (transpersonal therapies)

- any invasive or shocking holistic treatment

- catastrophic diets or catastrophic exercise regimens

These seem to be safe and I am glad to see re-emerging back into society and treatment:

- biofeedback and biofeedback devices.

- light bank therapy for seasonal depression (see www.toolsforwellness for winter lights and tapes and www.apolloheath.com for information on how to use and some newer types of seasonal depression lights. From the ApolloHealth web site, valuable information can also be found on biological rhythms that affect sleep and mood).

- relaxation tapes and CDs of any type; get many

- journals, journals, journals, unless your are too compulsive about it or a "manic writer"–those who cannot stop the flood of writing.

Family Participation

There may be questions of how involved a family should be with the mild moods. The answer is "always" for the bipolar 1s, and sometimes for soft bipolar.

However, some family members may not be willing to participate. Some have also become burned out with outlandish behavior or have been totally estranged.

Mood Charting

Mood charts help both the psychiatrist and the therapist. Mood charts should be brought to all treatment meetings, often kept in a three-ring notebook.

I prefer a simple, quickly drawn mood chart that may also track other issues, such as anxiety, sleep, and fearfulness. It just takes a minute each day to note on charts. There are standard mood charts available on the Internet. I don't find these too "consumer friendly" and helpful in tracking various issues for treatment.

Mood charting also allows a person to see changes in moods that they might not ordinarily be aware of. Mood charting can include records of life events. It increases insight about harmful things that cause mood cycling and activities that are beneficial.

Harmful stimuli:

drugs, alcohol

diets

not sleeping, or not sleeping within a regular schedule

overwork

getting run down, overextended, exhausted

over-the-counter medications without doctor's permission

trips and travel

illness

family conflict

holidays

getting too jazzed in the summer

obligation

life change, stress

death, illness in the family

getting married

getting divorced

Stabilizing Things:

sleep routines

taking medications regularly

making all therapy appointments

eating well

drinking water

exercise

rest

seeing friends, socializing

alone time, meditations

9

Medication and treatment specialists

Well, this might be the shortest chapter you've ever seen on medications and physicians for mood disorders, especially when you consider that it is *the foundational* treatment for the mood disorders.

But I have just found that the many books available on mood disorders have redundant and outdated chapters on the medications. Chances are, if you've seen one, you've seen them all. Most of the existing literature seems a bit gratuitous and not too consumer-friendly.

So, let me veer off the beaten track with a different approach. Let me guide you to the Internet resources you need to download current information on medications. This way, you'll always have the latest information right at your fingertips.

Most importantly, I tell my patients: my bipolar treatment programs, which are education and therapy for individuals and families, are for those persons *taking mood stabilizers*. I do not allow into the program those persons who:

- have not been properly evaluated for the disorder and diagnosed correctly.

- are not stable enough for the groups;

- do not understand the basics of how and why to take medications (usually need to completed 6-8 weeks of psychoeducation);

- are not seeing a general physician or psychiatrist strongly interested in treating mood disorders and are not being given appropriate supportive information from that person;

- are not rebelliously taking harmful over-the-counter medication, drinking or using illicit drugs.

The medications for the mild moods are similar to those used to treat the mood disorders.

For up-to-date and easy to read information, check out: www. psycheducation.org

For information specific medications, see: www.psycom.net

Information on new and experimental medications (such as Felbatol and Cere-byx), is available at: www.aafp.org/afe/980201/ap.curry.html

If you want to go very in-depth and see how and why physicians generally choose what medication to use, refer to the Expert Consensus Guideline Series, Treatment of Bipolar Disorder at http://www.psychguides.com/is a generic guide, and not followed by all Bipolar specialist physicians.

Doctors and Therapists

Finding a physician, psychiatrist, or therapist who is specialized and interested in treating bipolar disorder can be tough to do. But it is something you must do because poor treatment can either delay things or be disastrous.

To find these persons, you might call local mental health hotlines, hospital emergency rooms, and psychiatric clinics. Questions I would ask include:

What percentage of your practice is dedicated to mood disorders and the mild moods (cyclothymia)?

- What approach do you have to medications and side effects?

- What kind of education do you do in patient meetings?

- What is bipolar kindling and how do you address this?

Therapists include licensed clinical counselors, psychiatric social workers, and psychologists. You might ask them:

- What recent books and training have they completed on mood disorders?

- What percentage of their practice is dedicated to the mood disorders?

- What is their general interest in treating mood disorders?

- What model do they use in the treatment and do they have some minimal famil-iarity with IPRST and DBT, described earlier in this book?

- Do they work with a psychiatrist for symptom reporting if needed?

- Do they allow the family to be involved with treatment if appropriate?

10

Some questions

The mild moods have *many* questions when beginning treatment, especially when correcting years of bad treatment or years of emotional roller coastering. Again, I encourage using the book, *A Setback is a Setup for a Comeback* by Willie Jolley, as a foundation to "restart" or redirect your life. Take it slow. There's also great advice in the comic movie, *What About Bob*. Take baby steps.

Here are some common questions asked in the initial weeks of treatment.

Q. 1. I am just starting treatment and know that my current job is the wrong one for me. I feel very panicked to change now. What should I do?

A. Often, in any type of treatment we encourage individuals to wait on big decisions such as job changes or a divorce. You may want to get some career and work counseling before making a change. No matter what you do, a drastic change will only make things worse for now. Put up with things for a while so you can work with your psychiatrist and allow your medications to work. Medication changes alone are stressful.

Also, there is a saying: "Any decision made in panic will be a bad one." If you allow things to settle, your personal judgment should improve, and you should be better able to assess the work problem and run into needed opportunities. Take a deep breath, slow down, and take care of your mental health first.

Q. 2. The holidays are real triggers for me. I often get really wound up, and then upset. Nothing ever goes the way I hoped, and I don't even have any high expectations. Then, I am disappointed for months after. Is there any help?

A. The holiday season is very traumatic for many individuals. There is added stimulation of activities, foods, smells, etc. But suddenly we are pulled into all of our old ghosts of family, the past, and childhood, society and religious views. Whew!

The holiday season is particularly hard on the mild moods for these and other issues. Some can get wound up in flights of fun and activity, while others can spin downward in the somber coldness of hungry winter. It is just a time of extremes: feast or famine. And our bodies also take a toll from this season, reeling from waves of alcohol and cocktail-weenie-filled parties or days of punitive fasting diets. All of this contributes to instability, both physically and mentally.

I feel there is not enough said about the holidays. Mood disorder patients need to be well inoculated, prepared, for what is coming. The goal is that each person will make conscious choices for that season of what is in their best interest, particularly as a mild mood.

For a good reference on the various issues to look out for in the holiday season, take a look at *Holiday Blues: Rediscovering the Art of Celebration, a 12-month Guide to Getting Everything You Want out of Stressful Holidays and Family Gatherings* by Herbert Rappaport, Ph.D.

Here are some tips I pass out to bipolar patients during the holidays:

- Do less, slow down, prevent getting wound up.

- Stop, take a deep breath, and return back to yourself.

- Monitor your emotional levels daily.

- Keep foods routine. Don't skip meals. Diet only with your doctor's permission. Don't eat sugar treats without other foods. Carry some protein bars with you in case you are hungry.

- Run away fast from alcohol.

- Plan and organize what your want to participate in over the holidays: be in control of what happens to you.

- Journal, read, and continue all calming and centering practices.

- Watch out for spontaneous activities that might lead to being out late and skipping a night of sleep.

- Holidays often bring up old wounded memories; honor them but don't obsess or ruminate on past hurts.

- Drop expectations of yourself and others so you can flow with seasonal activities.

- Practice your sleep hygiene: routine habits and sleep times really help.

- Don't stop exercise. If you can't do routine exercise, get a short walk daily.

- Live out your own unique story for the holidays: don't ~~ety's ideas of what you ought to do. Refuse obligation.~~

- Plan to *not* do some activities.

- Don't skip medication. If you blew too much money on gifts, let your doctor's nurse know immediately if you are short on medication, and the two of you sort out a plan of action.

- Set limits on purchases; don't get into the "feeding frenzy" of shoppers in stores. Don't come out of stores with large bags of stuff and big bills. Don't even go into a store unless you have something specific to purchase. Don't make impulsive purchases. Don't buy a gift for a person and then later feel you didn't get enough and then buy a second and third gift. Consider gifts of favors, meals, nights out, etc. Don't give time-consuming crafts as gifts.

- Feel free to avoid uncomfortable situations.

- Don't get wound up before Christmas; a depressive crash will surely follow.

- Rent movies and do other calm, in-home activities with a few others.

- If you don't have a doctor's or therapist's appointment in December, at least call just before Christmas and a few days after just to leave a message of how you are doing. Have the nurse or therapist note this in your records.

- Don't get too many irons in the fire, too many projects started. Your bipolar treatment is based on managed and calm self-care.

Q. 3. I have been out of work for two years from depression, and have an intense fear of work. What steps might I take next?

A. I am sure that your fear is one that feels like a gigantic monster, sort of like some sort of life-threatening dragon that seemingly intends to destroy you or seemingly knows just how to work its ways on you. That's how our personal monsters are.

This fear of work can be pretty strong in the mild moods and mood disorders. It is likely that you do want to work, but that something keeps you from heading out the door to look for work. Others think it would be simple for you to make calls or fill out applications, but there may be terror associated with even these steps. You could begin with a work support group at your department of employment. Also, the metaphoric monster techniques mentioned in this book, will help page ____), if you keep working on them. Find a helpful friend, a supportive person, or a prayer partner. Use anything you can.

In treatment, we treat this problem like a phobia. One finds tools to calm anxiety while doing small projects to head to the bigger task. For instance, you would work on calming your fearful mind (the metaphor box), and panic responses in your body. At the same time, you might have a "step" plan to adjust to work.

Here is one person's step plan:

- Volunteer at the hospital two days per week, two months.

- Work two days per week, temp service.

- Work four days per week, temp service.

- Work half time in my line of work, six months.

- Seek full time work in my line of work.

Q. 4. I have a lot of anxiety going into public settings where others might look at me. Should I avoid them?

A. There is a high incidence of social phobias among the mood disorders. We know a lot about social phobias these days and how to treat them. We also know that if you face your fear in small amounts, you make headway.

But total avoidance can really lock you up. Sometimes the mood disorders get small episodes of agoraphobia, which is the fear of being away from safety or safe persons. At its worst, agoraphobics are afraid to leave their house.

Other common phobias are the fear of flying and the fear of public speaking. The mood disorders may have other odd and highly exaggerated phobias. I know several individuals terrified by moths, spiders, snakes, scorpions, and lizards. In each situation, the person experiences terrifying reactions just thinking about the events, and in the past had felt they were highly traumatized by contact. They had developed a form of post-traumatic stress disorder by their experience.

In traumatic phobia events, debriefing in therapy is required. Otherwise, highly behavioral work is very successful as described in Q. 3 above. This work, systematic desensitization, is lined out very well in *The Anxiety and Phobia Workbook* by Bourne.

Q. 5. I don't sleep well. Am I alone in this as a soft bipolar?

A. Many bipolars suffer from sleep problems and intrusive thoughts during insomnia. It is a serious matter as poor sleep leads to mood cycling. Work with your therapist on managing these intrusive thoughts.

You should also discuss this with your doctor. Overall, the mood disorders are known to not have good "body clocks." That is, there is no good internal mechanism that tells them when to sleep and wake like the rest of the population. So, they tend to be awake nights and sleep days. Parents of child mood disorders note this very early on.

While you and your doctor should work on this as a concern of treatment, there are things that you do that can keep you wound up and not sleep. Getting "wound up," and then not getting "wound down," in the evening contributes to poor sleep hygiene. Many people obsess about work or the next day and need to just put it aside. Those who are slightly manic may start working on projects and just forget to sleep, paying the price for several days.

Healthy sleep hygiene or habits may take years to acquire. Try these:

- Practice leaving work or chores with mental rituals at set times.

- Take a bath or sauna in evenings.

- Find reading that tends to wind you down (unless reading or certain types of reading jazz you up).

- Become aware of eating, medication, and exercise patterns—when you should do them so you can begin to wind down.

- Try to be aware of what is disturbing you at night so you can convey this to your doctor.

- Are you waking from sleep?

- Are outside noises waking you? Can you use earplugs?

- Is your mind racing? Or do you awaken in the morning with racing thoughts?

- Is your body electric, wired?

- Does your body hurt; are you feeling pain?

Check out "sleep hygiene" or "sleep disturbance" with Google Internet search engine. This is such an important topic and I hope that more information rises to the top for mood disorder patients on sleep disturbance. You will also find help-ful new research available on Bipolar Disorder and sleep regulation at: www.psycheducation.org/depression/clock.htm.

Some mood disorder patients use "gradual lights," which mimic the gradual onset of daylight, to turn on the daily body clock. You will find interesting arti-cles on this and support for this treatment among the mood disorders. To see the scope of sleep problems, refer to *Sleep Thieves: An Eye-Opener Exploration into the Science and Mysteries of Sleep* by Stanely Coren.

Q. 6. My boss seems just like me, a soft bipolar, and we really clash. How is it that I keep running into people like me?

A. It is very odd how we attract people much like ourselves. They say that opposites attract, but in reality, we seem to meet up with others who are like us, whether other alcoholics, others who were abused as children, or other mild moods.

I think these other people often serve as a good mirror or study of behavior for you. Usually, they are not in treatment. And you often don't have the opportu-nity to suggest that if it's your boss; be careful.

But you can see your own behavior, whether the mood shifts, the irritability, or family patterns. Many mild moods recount a history of having bosses and rela-tionships with characters where the mood disorders were present in mild form. Here, too, were people functional in the world, but with mood disturbances.

Carl Jung said that we keep running into these people to be further aware of our own inner issues. These persons are the necessary mirrors of our own behav-ior. That is something we sometimes don't like to admit to.

Q. 7. I come from a family of pretty bright cyclothymics, but none of us really met our potential. We always seemed to live on the "other side of the tracks." I see my personal potential, but know that there are several generations of history behind me. I am not a superhuman person who can overcome all this history. What can I do to reach my potential?

A. Indeed, this is a common story, and a sad one of the mild moods. All that CI (creative imagination) and no place to put it. Often, it just seems to go down to the gutter with a bottle of Jim Beam. It is especially for this reason that infor-mation and treatment of the mild moods must be brought forward. This should be the banner topic of this book.

Several generations of what society now just call's "issues" are hard to deal with. It is like you have your own person to carry around in life, say just about your height. But then, you have this toady, sneaky dude or dudette dogging you—your shadow. This person following you is not as big as you are, metaphorically speaking. Let's say he or she is a foot shorter. But they are there at every turn, telling you whether or not you will succeed or fail in a job, relationship, weight loss, or even the minutest issue in your life. This is the judge and jury of your life.

Some call this the "family shadow." Others call this the "old contaminating parent." Whatever you call it, it is wrong, and not needed. Find a way through a therapist, a support group (*Course in Miracles*, ACOA, ACA), or a book, (such as *Embracing the Inner Critic: Turning Self-Criticism into a Creative Asset* by Hal and Sidra Stone), to whack this on the head.

This family shadow character will daily try to sneak back, moment by moment. This is because this "issue" is deeply ingrained in your psyche. You will have to find a daily method of honoring, yet stopping, this role—yes, for life. I suggest to many persons, once they recognize the inner critic, to find a small action figure at a store that could represent this issue. Put it on your bureau, and honor it, but metaphorically, leave it on the bureau daily.

There is much written about what is called the "impostor syndrome," where a person feels like an impostor, but may have a successful job. Another twist to this is the "underearner," a person internally successful, but often underpaid in jobs. Both problems are issues of low self esteem. The latter problem is discussed in the book *Earn What You Deserve* by Jerrold Mundis.

Q. 8. I have tried medication for the mild moods and am still having panic and mood shifts. It is not working. Have I failed treatment?

A. Keep a chart of your anxiety and moods. Take this to your doctor. Sometimes people underrate the severity of the mood disorders in their life and among family members. Then, the doctor needs to address this as bipolar 1 or 2, and treat it appropriately. There is no failure of treatment, only feedback. Medical treatment can be very different for each person and that is why you want to see a mood disorder specialist.

Q. 9. I am getting better on my mood stabilizer, but I am sure I traumatized my new wife of this last six months with my rapid mood swings. What should we do about that?

A. Discuss this with your doctor or therapist in a meeting with your wife. Sometimes, there is a benefit in the initial stages to have a private meeting with the spouse if that person may have been traumatized. They may have developed depression or if in the relationship for a while, even developed some form of trauma disorder. No matter how this happens, I think it is important to recognize that the spouse is often the co-victim of the disorder and will have also developed problems out of this.

Personally, I try to get the spouse into the family member support group and then screened by their own family physician for depression. While starting mild moods in therapy, too many types of therapy services too soon may burn them out or frighten them or cause monumental costs. Getting the mild mood stabilized and the spouse screened for depression, though, is a priority.

You ought to sit down and ask your spouse how their experience went this last year. It is possible that you actually were like some sort of mood steam roller or amusement ride they unwittingly got on. If you need to polish up your listening skills, review the book *The Lost Art of Listening: How Learning to Listen Can Improve Relationships* by Michael P. Nichols, Ph.D.

Q. 10. I was diagnosed five years ago and tried the medications. They didn't work for me. I want to go to the treatment group, but your require members to take mood stabilizers. This is unfair.

A. Things have changed in the last few years. Doctors have many mood stabilizers to choose from and can assist you in finding one that will not have the bad side effects that turned you off previously. You can collaborate with your doctor on this. I urge you to try medication again.

Q. 11. I have a deep dread of Sunday nights. It hits about 3 p.m. and escalates. It is like the cloud of death. I can't get rid of it. I know it is about my work concerns.

Some fears and issues for mood disorders can be deep and very visceral. That is the down side of CI. If this pattern has gone on for years, it can be really tough to crack.

If you have just started treatment, I would try various methods to try to intervene with the problem. Certainly, this is a brain lock, and you might want to look into EMDR, eye movement desensitization reprocessing, a method of unlocking thoughts in the brain. There are books on how to do this yourself, and there are therapists who specialize it.

Inform your physician about this, also. There are medications to be recommended for this. Keep track of these thoughts on a calendar, ranking the severity of the event on a scale of 1 to 10 so that you can report this to your doctor.

Q. 12. I went to a bipolar support group, but they were not taking mood-stabilizing medication. Should I go back?

A. No. There is too much difference between those in the three camps: those on mood stabilizers, those on the wrong medications, and those religiously on herbs or resisting treatment. It creates a sort of war zone and you don't want to be there!

Q. 13. My doctor says I have "hysteroid dysphoria." What is this?

A. Dysphoria is the exact opposite of euphoria; instead of being elated, you are intensely down. The current term used for this is hyperthymic depression. This is where the person is depressed, but there is still an abundance of emotion and thought, albeit, painful.

Obviously, you feel intensely bad, and should not feel intensely bad about a diagnosis. It is just part of the mild moods. There are other disorders that share the problems of intensity of pain. There are needs to:

- validate yourself;

- calm yourself;

- remind yourself of worth, your life, direction, and goals;

- keep small daily tasks on track.

You might enjoy all the wealth of knowledge from some other "pain cousins," those who have fibromyalgia. You can find online the magazine *Fibromyalgia Aware* and they will send you a free sample copy.

Again, you should discuss the pain of this with your doctor, as there are medications to treat this.

Q. 14. I am feeling odd things in my body, like hot and cold. I don't want my psychiatrist to think I am too nutty. Should I share this?

A. I have found that those doctors with true interest in the mood disorders are highly interested in any symptoms and medication side effects you may feel. Simply make a list called "odd body feelings" and share this with your doctor. Besides, wouldn't it be nice to get some relief? That's what the doctor is there for. Don't hide from him or her the very thing that you'd like to be relieved of.

Q. 15. I feel I lost 15 years in time due to the wrong diagnosis. I was diagnosed as having panic disorder. Now, I am on track, but what should I do with the grief?

A. Well, you have lost 15 years. So there is certainly some grief to be dealt with. Perhaps with a therapist or friend you would like to recount a history of what was lost, and complete some ceremony. Maybe place the story on the shelf and symbolically step over some threshold representing your move to a new life.

Whatever you do, you will want to do something to mark the event that you can remember. However, if you fail to do so, you could risk wallowing in grief for many years, and that, too, would be another loss in your life.

Consider also the opposite side. What, precisely, were the benefits gained from those 15 years of experience? Wisdom? Depth of character? Broad life experience? Patience? Find at least one thing to be grateful for regarding that time, and regarding the disorder.

You might like the book, *Dark Night of the Soul: A Guide To Finding Your Way Through Life's Ordeals,* by Thomas Moore. In this book, Moore discusses the many metaphoric purposes of dark times in our life. Just like Jonah and the whale, a crisis or hard time spits us up on some necessary beach, later. These hard times are times of incubation, birthing, and change. Three metaphoric movies of this are *The Legend of Bagger Vance, The Wizard of Oz,* and *Hook.*

Q. 16. What can I do to stabilize my weight and diet?

A. Some medications cause weight gain and others are neutral. Weight is an issue to track and often discuss with your doctor.

But what can you do to help? Simply put, the mood disorders benefit from a diet that is very stable, but not necessarily bland. Those diets that promote stable blood sugar seem to promote stable mood. These include the Zone diet, any diabetic diet, and the brand new Hampton diet.

Conversely, those diets that promote unstable blood sugar also promote mood swings. These include the Atkins diet or any carb-free diet (ketogenic diets cause mania and impact some mood stabilizers), any radical diet, or any protein-free diet.

Routine exercise is a very important topic that I bring up in mental health groups. I often recommend:

• scheduled exercise

• reading books on exercise

- reporting exercise on mood charts

- seeing a trainer if you need help getting going

- yoga or Tai Chi

- walking

- not getting extreme; don't overdo it

One book that may have advantages for those who have not exercised in the past is the book, *The Step Diet: Count Calories To Lose Weight And Keep It Off Forever*, by Pamela Peeke. This book is not about dieting at all, but about using a pedometer to count your steps taken daily.

Some soft bipolars are just awful with eating habits, the worst problem being just forgetting to eat at all. Some even skip drinking water. Not eating leads to mood swings.

Q. 17. I am pretty disorganized and also get stressed easily. What should I do?
Stress and its impact on the bipolar sufferer are often not addressed. It does contribute to mood cycling and a host of bad behaviors. Consider these helpful books:

- *The Idiot's Guide to Organizing your Life*, by Georgene Lockwood

- *TimeLock: How Life Got So Hectic and What you Can Do About It*, by Ralph Keyes

- *The End of Stress as We Know t*, by Bruce McEwen

- *Urgency Addiction: How to Slow Down Without Sacrificing Success*, by Nina Tassi, Ph.D

- *The 10 Natural Laws of Successful Time and Life Management: Proven Strategies for Increased Productivity and Inner Peace*, by Hyrum W. Smith (creator of the Franklin day planner)

- *Personal Time Management*, by Marion F. Haynes

- *The Time Bind: When Work Becomes Home and Home Becomes Work*, by Arlie Russell Hochschild

You might also want to seek out a personal or life coach to get organized if that is needed to keep a business or other venture on track. You can find personal coaches on the Internet or through your local Chamber of Commerce.

Q. 18. With all these mood shifts, I would like to be more mindful of myself, connected with my inner foundation. What would you recommend?

A. Mindfulness and centerdness are not trendy words for mild moods, but important ones. Each person needs to find methods that fit them personally and also fit their culture. You may want to contact your church or a spiritual advisor on methods of centering that might work for you. There are many useful and helpful books on mindfulness and centerdness at your favorite bookseller.

Several patients have recommended the books, *The Power of Now*, by Echart Tolle; *Loving What Is*, by Byron Katie; *Help Yourself*, by Dave Pelzer and *A Setback is a Setup for a Comeback*, by Willie Jolley

Not every book is for everyone. Journaling, daily ritual, and prayer are "transcultural" and fit 99 percent of persons on the planet. I think that the mild mood people are highly spiritual and benefit from encouragement in this area in their life. Being mindful and centered is a wonderful way to have greater stability in your life and thereby allow your medications to work, let alone opening up its own treasure trove of inner life riches.

Q. 19. What is "chipping away?"

A. Chipping away is a term borrowed from the field of alcoholism and chemical dependency treatment. In chipping away, a recovering person chips away at a solid recovery base, like taking a hatchet to a tree. If they miss meetings, allow bad habits to return, or don't do follow-up care, the tree's trunk is "chipped away" at, but each small chip, ever so small, leads to the big fall.

So, too, mood disorder patients need to watch for chipping away behavior and attitudes that lead to a fall or relapse. This can include thoughts, attitudes, and behaviors that lead to the relapse, or return to square one. Unfortunately for the mood disorder patients, each fall becomes more severe as actual mild damage to brain tissue becomes accumulative. Chipping away can include:

- drinking alcohol

- not monitoring sleep or food patterns

- not making therapy meetings, canceling or delaying appointments

- skipping medication

- not taking the disorder seriously

- believing others why they discount or stigmatize the mood disorders

- not filling prescriptions

- not doing any recovery project

- falling back into any old bad habit

- not conveying information to therapist or psychiatrist

- using over-the-counter medication, marijuana, or illicit drugs

- using steroids

- not letting a spouse or relative give feedback on symptoms

- not charting moods if they have been asked to do so

- getting too busy

- justifying something, blaming

- not reporting mild mania or other symptoms

- unconscious sabotaging

Q. 20. What is bipolar kindling?

A. I am including this concise and critical article on kindling.

"If a bipolar person goes untreated for a period of years, could he or she begin to experience rapid cycling or become treatment-resistant? If stressors initially set off episodes, in time, could episodes appear without any such triggers? Research says the answer to all these questions is yes, and the reason may be a process that has been termed 'kindling.'

"The phenomenon of kindling in epilepsy was first discovered by accident by researcher Graham Goddard in 1976. Goddard was studying the learning process in rats, and part of his studies included electrical stimulation of the rats' brains at a very low intensity, too low to cause any type of confusion. What he found was that after a couple of weeks of this treatment, the rats did experience confusion when the stimulation was applied. Their brains had become sensitized to electricity, and even months later, one of these rats would convulse when stimulated (History, 1998). Goddard and others later demonstrated that it was possible to induce kindling via chemicals as well (Hargreaves, 1996.)

"The name "kindling" was chosen because the process was likened to a log fire. The log itself, while it might be suitable fuel for a fire, is very hard to set afire in the first place. But surround it with small, easy to light pieces of wood–kindling–and set these blazing, and soon the log itself will catch fire.

"Dr. Robert M. Post of the National Institute of Mental Health (USA) is credited with first applying the kindling model to bipolar disorder (NARSAD). Demitri and Janice Papolos, in their excellent book, *The Bipolar Child*, describes this model as follows:

'…initial periods of cycling may begin with an environmental stressor, but if the cycles continue to occur unchecked, the brain becomes kindled or sensitized–pathways inside the central nervous system are reinforced…'

"Thus, many researchers now believe that kindling contributes to both rapid cycling and treatment resistant bipolar disorder. In addition, cocaine and alcohol have their own kindling effects, which can contribute to bipolar kindling.

"What does this mean for the bipolar patient? Take your medications as prescribed. Stopping treatment now could make your condition actually worsen and become more difficult to treat in the future.

"If you have not been diagnosed, but feel you may be manic-depressive, seek treatment, the sooner the better.

"Be honest with your prescribing doctor if you have an alcohol or drug problem, so he or she can evaluate your medication therapy accordingly." (http:// Bipolar.about.com/com/health/Bipolar/library/weekly/aa000917a.htm)

In addition to this information on kindling, the SSRI antidepressants have also been found to cause kindling. www.neurotransmitter.net/admania.html

This brings up the important issue of drinking and drug use. I am not a puritanical person. It is just that for the mood disorder persons, these chemicals wreak havoc on brain chemistry. For instance, to get really "soused" at a barbecue, you might suffer as a mood disorder person in three ways:

• There is the immediate impact on the brain from the hangover, and a disruption in your schedule in time of taking your medication. This could disrupt mood stability and biorhythms and take four to five days to recover from.

• There is latent mood cycling that comes into play three to seven days after. People just don't know where the mania or depression comes from when all else is going well, but this is cycling started by shifted brain chemistry. What you did on the weekend shows up several days later.

• Ongoing drinking or drug use causes kindling, which causes scarring of brain tissue, which causes either mania or rapid cycling. Patients often justify heavy pot use as recreation, or party drugs, or a weekend of cocaine in Las Vegas as just fun, but the damage is done, and it takes the brain months or years to recover.

Q. 21. I don't want to take medication. Why?

A. The three top reasons mild moods do not want to take medications are stigma, the "sirens' call," and loss of self control.

Stigma—There is a feeling that if they take medication such as the mood stabilizers, they will be seen as mental, or broken.

Others have difficulty adjusting to the chronic nature of the mood disorders. Medications are taken daily long-term, as they just don't seem to go away. It may feel or actually look like they are symptom free for months at a time, but the rule of thumb is that they just "cycle" back.

The sirens' call—Some do not want to leave their own sense of control and personal normalcy of the disorder. They have become familiar with the symptoms and may have developed a lifestyle of many years of coping mechanisms to deal with them. It might be very comfortable and safe to be mildly depressed, hypomanic, or chaotic and cycling.

On the other hand, there are certain threats to the stability of moods:

What would I do, or who would I be, if I were not depressed?

What would others think of me if I were not bubbly all the time?

What would I do, or who would I be, without chaos in my life?

My life if based on fear; how would I face a normal world of vacations and shopping at the mall if I took medication?

Also, there are those who have the sirens' call that is just the call of attraction to the darker, more evil, side of the mood.

Jeff admitted that he would not go on medication because he occasionally experienced the euphoria of mild mania and nobody was going to take that sensation buzz away from him.

Betty was involved in a Goth group, loved her dark poetry, and was known for her dark and morbid views of life. She had come to like being sullen and found her personality had become deeply wrapped up with her depressive nature. She feared treatment would change that and she did not know how she would make adjustments to her world.

In these cases, successful treatment will also be dependent in helping the individuals to deal with "intrapsychic" issues that would otherwise cause them to stop treatment. In facilitating adjustment, the person can find ways to both recover from the brain disorder and find mood stability, while making meaningful adjustments in their lives.

Impaired awareness of illness can also come from damage to specific parts to the brain for bipolar and schizophrenia patients who do not take their medication. For a complete review of impaired awareness of the illness, check out the legal briefing paper complete with research and court cases at http:// wwwpsychlaws.org/BriefingPapersBP14htm

Loss of Self-Control—Most mood disorder sufferers have a relationship with their mood problem based on years of coping, ruminating, fleeing, running, or whatever. It is like living with a comic sidekick in some TV sitcom. You're irritated with them, but don't want to get rid of them. And most of all, you don't want anyone to upset the progressive drama or story that they have going with you.

Mood disorder sufferers feel that both medications and therapy upset what they have had control of—that peaceful mood chaos in their mind

What? Couldn't make sense of this one?

Addressing and discussing why we resist medication or therapy is how we address these three common concerns.

Appendix A

Soft bipolar symptom self report

Do you or any family members have any of the following?

- alcoholism, such as binge drinking, daily drinking, or drinking to alleviate other symptoms or life problems

- anxiety or panic attacks

- behavioral addictions or compulsions, such as shopping, gambling, cleaning, eating, internet surfing or chat rooms, or sexual

- child abuse or spousal abuse, including verbal attacks or throwing things

- chronic aches and pains, or Arthritic-like symptoms (fibromyalgia, chronic fatigue syndrome), digestive problems, or other frequent illnesses, which truly do exist (somatic illness)

- chronic headaches or migraines

- chronic Irritability, or not irritable at work but irritable at home

- mild legal problems such as getting speeding tickets or other "tests" of the law, or severe legal problems such as incarceration

- depression in childhood

- depression in the winter

- drug abuse or drug addiction, including use of marijuana

- eccentric or unusual behavior

- extreme worry, obsessiveness and compulsiveness

- frequent depression, in episodes, in the week, or even times of day

- hypersensitivity to light, noises, touch, crowds, etc.

- mood swings, shifts in energy

- if a woman, post-partum depression or post-partum psychosis

- reactive/destructive

- religious addiction or religious compulsions

- sleep disorders, unable to sleep or extensive sleeping

- suicide or suicide threats, including severe feelings of hopelessness

- talking continually, talking fast

- unusual reactions to prescription medications, hypersensitivity to medications

- vivid and unusual fears, extreme childhood nightmares

- withdrawal or agoraphobic behaviors

- history of work, social, or relationship problems

- a prior diagnosis of bipolar disorder, borderline personality disorder, or a psychiatric hospitalization

- have two or more psychiatric diagnoses, such as panic, depression, or some other anxiety

- take antidepressants and felt odd immediately, or feel well immediately, or the antidepressants have a pattern of failing in benefit after a few months

- use various over-the-counter remedies to treat anxiety, sleep problems, mood problems, etc.

- seem bright, but not meeting potential

- get stuck on a thought, issue, or feeling and can't move on

- have moods, emotions, or a lifestyle that seems different or more extreme than the average person

- known for some trait, such as being keyed up, withdrawn, a meddler, bubbly, hyperactive, energetic, irritable, or volatile

Do you have varying periods of:

- sharpened and creative thinking alternating with periods of mental confusion and apathy

- good mood versus times of low or irritable mood

- loss of interest or pleasure versus elevated and expansive mood

- decreased need for sleep versus too much need for sleep

- shaky self esteem and lack of self confidence versus naïve grandiose overconfidence

- unusual work hours with much done versus periods of down time and recuperation

- more uninhibited people seeking or social good times versus introverted self-absorption or withdrawal from others

- involvement in pleasurable activities versus restricted involvement in pleasurable actives and feelings of guilt over past activities

- optimism or exaggeration of past achievement versus pessimistic attitude toward the future or brooding about past events

- more talkative than usual with laughing, joking, and punning versus less talkative with tearfulness or crying

- financial extravagance versus periods of guilt and self punishment

- more sexual or impulsive versus over-constraint or held-back

- shopping, spending, and doing versus low activity

- feeling in slow motion versus feeling in fast motion.

- feeling serious or morbid versus happy

- feeling like your body is heavy or you feel old versus feeling light or energetic

- feeling aware of the outer world versus feeling introspective and that others are looking at you

- feeling resourceful and having ideas versus feeling stuck and limited

- having strong or increased body senses and sensations versus feeling everything is dull, tasteless, and boring

- feeling free to live in the world and society versus feeling you live in your head and are stuck with painful feelings, especially guilt and self-criticism

Characteristics of the "up" state

These are extensive lists: not all characteristics fit all persons: thank goodness!

In the up feeling state, do you have any of these traits?

cheerful

exuberant

optimistic

self aware

boastful

energetic

versatile

stimulus seeking

short sleeper

irritable

happy

enhanced senses

increased intelligence

distracted

accelerated thoughts

decreased inhibitions

increased libido

feel good physically

start projects

excessive

fast.

colorful

flamboyant

social

like noise and stimulation

do several things at once

negligent driving

increased appetite

others seen in slow motions

spending

poor judgment

itching

greater sensitivity

increased alcohol or tobacco use

feel hot

mild euphoria

excessive writing

vivid imagery

vivid tastes

controlled by the present fun or future ideas in harmful way

humorous, likes dating and comedy

may be the life of the party but scares others off

elaborate

charm

would rather talk

lose money, resources

has open boundaries with others

increased alcohol and caffeine intake, including rapid intake of same

inappropriate or loud laughter

reading or doing several projects at one time, multitasking

eat rapidly or forget to eat at all

engrossed in projects and may forget to drink water or go to bathroom

too much dreaming of the future, inventions, money making, lottery, etc.

disregard time or needs of others

vulnerable to other high risk behaviors

may anxiously take care of personal needs such as household needs or personal grooming

may be excessively helpful with neighbors, relatives, or strangers, whether they request help or not

do projects that are "off track" and may not support true goals or income needs

excessive punning, jokes, risky or vulgar language

Soft bipolar depression

On the down, depressed side, symptoms and behaviors can, but don't always, include:

gloomy

humorless, avoids comedy and dating

guilt

sluggish

slow, passive

devoted

long sleep

anxiety

panic

self-deprecation

unexplained fears

lethargic, feels drained

morbid preoccupation

lowered consciousness

lowered output

decreased verbal output

less talk

withdrawal

mental confusion

memory problems

tearfulness

self-absorbed

ruminative or stuck thoughts

feel dull

skeptical or paranoid

compulsions

lack of interests

may feel ill or sick

overwhelmed by stimulus

feel cold

vivid dark images

go to a dark place

indecision

heavy heart, burdened

foggy, feels like a mist, inability to focus

Feels heavy, leaden arms or legs

sore, tired, may have many illnesses (somatic illness)

suicidal or hopeless thoughts

paranoid or fearful of others

fault finding of others

may worry about others or start codependency patterns

rumination on past, flood of melancholy feelings

avoid responding to phone messages, email, and responsibilities

feel there are no options, stuck, trapped

feel left alone by others, alone in life, different than others

time is lost and not productive, free time is often not utilized well

has sudden and almost complete loss of goals, direction, focus, and self esteem

overwhelmed by responsibility, paperwork, bills, etc.

want left alone, feels need to back out of prior commitments

feel personally empty, bankrupt, that personal needs are not and will not be met

feel others have unfair advantage and are not "broken" like you

procrastinate

vulnerable to others, is pushed over by others

may escape for hours or days in television, an old hobby, books, or other pastime that is solitary

may not take care of self, household, personal needs

may give up on social projects or obligations to help others or family

prone to eat fatty or other foods known to be bulky or not nutritious (less carb craving, more fat craving)

feel rejected by others, overly sensitive, feelings on shoulders

abrupt and sharp with others, may not realize it until later

discouraging toward own self

Mixed state (depression and anxiety at the same time)

agitation

feeling disorganized

irritation

worry

feeling something is going to happen

feeling tired, but may need to pace

apprehension

dysphoria, not feeling good, which is just the opposite of a feeling of euphoria, and this can be pretty bad for the mixed-states, including going on for weeks or years

can't sleep, tired during the day

depressed mood

rapid thoughts

lack of flexibility

may perseverate (hyper-focus) on some issue because of internal anxiety and fear: can't get off a topic can't wait

intense responses to any perceived or biological stressor

rigid responses or needs

oppositional

carb craving

distractible, seems like has attention deficit hyperactive disorder

separation anxiety

may be more prone to impulsive or addictive behaviors during this time

edgy, may even fidget or pace

may seem bothersome or irritate spouse or relatives

obsessive and compulsive

Appendix B

Mood Disorder Screening Tool©

For family physicians, gynecologists, nurses, counselors, and social workers

One percent of the population suffers from severe bipolar mood disorder (manic-depressive disorder). However, up to another three percent of the population suffers from other forms of the mood disorders. Approximately one-fourth of those with unipolar depression actually have unipolar-bipolar depression, and one-fifth of women who experience depressive or psychotic post-partum depression are experiencing the opening of bipolar mood disorder.

The Mood Disorder Screening Tool (MDST) is based on new insights on the whole spectrum of mood disorders present in the population, including milder form, soft bipolar. New classifications of mood disorders have been suggested that do not fit the understanding of typical manic and depressive cycles. Those suggested types are:

- type 1 mania and depression.

- type 2 hypomania (milder mania) and Depression.

- type 3 cyclothymia (mild mania followed by mild depression, with mood shifts often caused by life events, there is no spontaneous hypomania).

- type 4 hypomania or mania precipitated by medication (particularly antidepressants and illicit drugs).

- type 5 depressed patients with bipolar relatives or depressed patients with alcoholic parents.

- type 6 mania without depression.

- hyperthymia (florid thoughts, fears, emotions, nightmares, vivid daydreams, often with "happy and social" mood).

- hyperthymic depression (florid thoughts, fears, emotions, with "pained," depressed mood).

- (types 1-4 from Gerald Klerman, MD, 1987; another list calls bipolar 3 depression without hypomania with Hyperthymia Akiskal, 1983)

The Mood Disorder Screening Tool is not a complete diagnostic tool, but quickly screens individuals are at risk of misdiagnosis or harm from inappropriate medications. Positive responses should be followed by further diagnostic exploration. The MDST is especially useful in screening all patients prior to prescribing antidepressants, because they may be related to:

- manic or hypomanic responses to the SSRI antidepressants.

- patient switching from a stable bipolar disorder to more severe.

- actual scarring of brain tissue, exacerbating the mood disorder for life.

- decrease in long term compliance with treatment due to bad medication responses.

See "SSRI Induced Mania/Rapid Cycling Research, Articles, and Links" www.neurotransmitter.net/admania.html.

Remember: 40 percent of bipolar patients attempt suicide and 20 percent complete their attempt.

Mood Disorder Screening Tool©

Please check off in the right-hand columns if any of these characteristics apply. In the first column, place a mark if it applies to you. In the second column, place a mark if it applies to any blood-relative of yours. Place a check in the question column if you are uncertain for any reason that the question might possibly apply to you or your relative.

Please do not rush through the questions. You should complete this in a place where you are not distracted because your responses are important. If you do not understand any question or need help on any part, feel free to ask for assistance from the person who gave you this form.

The estimated time it will take you to complete this is less than 10 minutes.

Question	me	relative	not sure
1. Is there a prior diagnosis of Bipolar Disorder, mood disorder, psychosis, schizophrenia, borderline personality, a hospitalization for any of these, or depression or anxiety?	/	\	
2. Have you ever been prescribed mood stabilizers or antipsychotic medication (such as lithium, Depakote, Gabatril, Trileptal, Neurontin, Haldol, Risperidal, Zyprexa, or others)?	x		x mom
3. Have you ever been told you have various psychiatric disorders (such as depression, general anxiety, panic, obsessive-compulsive disorder, borderline personality, psychotic disorder, schizophrenia, Bipolar Disorder, etc.), or that you have had several of these at different periods of time?	no		x
4. Have you had depression or anxiety and needed more than one medication at a time?	X		
5. If you ever took an antidepressant, did you: initially feel odd, unreal or anxious or agitated, have an almost immediate improvement, stop the medication from some odd reaction, or take antidepressants and find that they stopped working after a while?	X		
6. Did you have a pattern of childhood depression, fears, or anxiety?	X		
7. Women only: did you have a reaction after the birth of a child that was termed post-partum depression or post-partum psychosis?	no		
8. Have you ever had suicidal thoughts or feelings, or attempted suicide?	X		
9. Have you ever had periods of elation, euphoria, extreme energy, risk-taking, lessened need for sleep, racing thoughts, or starting many projects at the same time?	X		

	M	R	NS
10. Have you ever had periods of depression, lethargy, lack of interest, hopelessness, inability to think or solve problems, or slowed physical motions (sluggish and uncoordinated)?	X	X	
11. Have you or others noted that you have mood swings?	X	X	
12. Have you ever been depressed and felt anxious or agitated at the same time?	X		
13. Have you had periods where you have had problems with impulsiveness, overeating, gambling, shopping, or any other compulsive behavior?	X	X	
14. Have you had periods of extreme interest in sex or periods with lack of interest in sex?	X		
15. Have you had in childhood or adulthood vivid fears, vivid emotions, realistic nightmares, or realistic "daytime dreams"?	X		
16. Do you have vivid physical or emotional pain, heightened sensitivity to sensations such as noise or light, which may cause you pain or to withdraw from others or the world?			
17. Do you have ongoing or repeated work, social, or family problems?	X		
18. Do you use regularly or binge on alcohol, use marijuana or other illicit drugs, or use over-the-counter medications to treat emotional or sleep problems?			
19. Are you known as irritable or reactive and often criticize yourself or others, start arguments, have fights, or throw things during an emotional upset?	X		
20. Are you concerned that your bad thoughts and feelings are not normal, could be harmful, or could get worse?	X		

Appendix C

10-point physician bipolar disorder quick screen

Before you prescribe an antidepressant

(Antidepressants prescribed for bipolar depression can backfire, causing mania in the short term and worsening of the Bipolar 1llness in the long term (see www.neurotransmitter.net/admania.html). This is a liability issue and should be taken seriously.

Does the patient have:

A prior history of Bipolar Disorder l, ll or lll?
A family history of Bipolar Disorder?
A history of childhood depression?
A history of these reactions to prior antidepressant treatment: immediate "brightening," immediate recovery, bizarre or manic reactions?
A history of prior antidepressant treatment where the medication stops efficacy after a few months and the patient is again depressed on the antidepressant?
Untreatable adult depression?
Mood or energy cycles (low mood versus elevated mood [hypomanic: gregarious and energetic, or typical manic])?
Multiple psychiatric diagnoses, such as depression, phobias, anxiety disorders, personality disorders, etc.?
Post-partum depression or psychosis?
Addictions, compulsions, obsessions, eating disorders?

US Copyright August 25, 2004. Reproduction or Transmission is Prohibited. To register for clinical use go to: www.MoodDisorder.net

Appendix D

Samples of three methods to list or chart moods and different symptoms

You can design one yourself and take to each doctor's and therapist's visit.

Individualized weekly symptom report

Use the Soft Bipolar Symptom list to generate your own list of symptoms that represent your mood states. Use your list to graph your mood and anxiety. Also, complete this weekly and take this and your mood chart to all therapist and psychiatrist meetings.

My symptoms   strength of the symptom

(5 is strongest)

                                        1   2   3   4   5

Up mood state

1.

2.

3.

4.

5.

Mixed state

1.

2.

3.

4.

5.

Down mood state

1.

2.

3.

4.

5.

Your suicidal thoughts or para-suicidal thoughts or actions this last week (always report any suicidal or homicidal thoughts to your mental health specialist at once):

Example 2

Joan's homemade mood chart shows mood, anxiety and some other issues she is tracking.

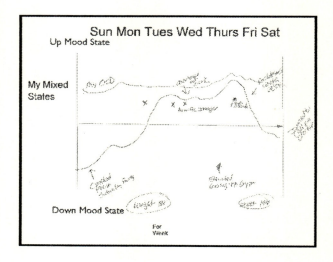

Example 3

Personalized Symptom mood/anxiety chart
Name:

symptom
Markers
5 each state

► **Week of** _____

►	Sun	Mon	Tue	Wed	Thu	Fri	Sat
►5							
►4							
►3							
►2							
►1							
►0							
►-1							
►-2							
►-3							
►-4							
►-5							
►							

► Other life events or notes:
► Medications taking:
► Did you take medications as prescribed?

If you are having a serious problem, call your local hospital, local mental health emergency hotline or National Suicide Hotline 1-800-784-2433

Teens: Girl's and Boys Town National Hotline 1-800-448-3000

Coming some time this summer will be the book, *More on Soft Bipolar*, covering:

- working with the inner creator, problem solver, and protector
- intrusive thoughts: ruminating
- intrusive thoughts: fears and panic
- intrusive thoughts when you have insomnia
- working with your warning signs and mood triggers
- relaxation and calming practice
- daily practices to help yourself
- mindfulness
- health and the soft bipolar
- rebuilding your life

A final note: Good luck to you in finding information, direction, and hope with your Soft Bipolar mild mood disorder! Charles K. Bunch, Ph.D.

978-0-595-34824-
0-595-34824-6

Printed in the United States
35854LVS00006B/34